HYPERACTIVE

HYPERACTIVE

THE CONTROVERSIAL HISTORY OF ADHD

Matthew Smith

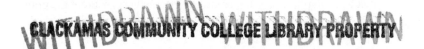
REAKTION BOOKS

To my mother, who always stuck up for me,
and to Dashiell, who bounced his way through
the writing of this book

Published by Reaktion Books Ltd
33 Great Sutton Street
London EC1V 0DX, UK

www.reaktionbooks.co.uk

First published 2012

Printed and bound in Great Britain
by TJ International, Padstow, Cornwall

British Library Cataloguing in Publication Data
Smith, Matthew, 1973–
Hyperactive : the controversial history of ADHD
1. Attention-deficit hyperactivity disorder – History.
2. Attention-deficit hyperactivity disorder – Etiology.
3. Attention-deficit hyperactivity disorder – Treatment – History.
I. Title
618.9'28589–dc23

ISBN: 978 1 78023 031 3

Contents

Preface

Historians do not have to have a personal connection to what they research, but when they do, it is appropriate that it is laid bare to be examined. If one picks up a social history of Britain, it is helpful to know if the author has ties to a particular political party. If one is reading a history of Israel, the author's opinions about the building of new Israeli settlements could be pertinent. And if one is reading about the history of medicine, especially by a historian who is interested in placing the history of health and medicine in its cultural, social and political contexts, it is appropriate that the context of my own investigations is revealed. So, why am I interested in hyperactivity?

I was not aware of such a thing growing up and going to school in the 1980s. I remember problem kids, and might have even been one on occasion, but never recalled such boys or girls being referred to as hyperactive, or being labelled with any other disorder. Bad kids were simply bad kids, at least as far as I was concerned. Attending school during the years in which disabled children were being included in mainstream classrooms, I do remember children who we, and the teachers, referred to as 'retarded', but none of these children seemed particularly hyperactive. I know now that many of these children had either Down's Syndrome, were suffering from a brain injury or were seriously learning disabled. There is also a story told in my family of my mother being sat down during a parent-teacher interview when I was in kindergarten, and being told that I had a learning disability on the grounds that I could not use scissors properly and had difficulties staying upright on a balance beam.

This did not go over well with my mom and I began grade one in a different school, where my learning disability, so-called, remained forever hidden.

Instead, the first hyperactive kid I met knowingly, I met as an adult. He sticks out in my memory for many reasons, not least because we shared a first name and he looked a little bit like I did at his age, which was about six or seven. I was a nervous student teacher at a middling primary school; he was one of my students. And there was no question that he was an active little boy. If he had his druthers, I am confident that Matthew would have happily bounced around the classroom, sharpening his pencil, looking out the window, trying on all the other kids' boots, investigating what was kept in the corner cupboard and generally doing his best impression of a perpetual motion machine from the time of the principal's welcoming address on the PA system to the dinging of the home-time bell. It was as if sitting at his desk quietly was ana-thema to him, an abhorrent condition to be avoided at all cost.

I have to admit that, when I was in charge of the classroom, Matthew's escapades did not annoy me a great deal. He tended not to bother the other kids terribly much and, while roaming around the room did not help him complete his work, neither did forcing him to sit in his seat. Sternly ordering Matthew to remain seated at his desk merely generated an impressive and, to all but the sternest pedagogue, amusing set of contortions in the boy as he found ways to balance his chair on one of its legs, while keeping only the index finger of one hand in contact with his desk. He could follow instructions, it appeared, just his own interpretation of them. But while I was content to let him do his thing, finding a few minutes when possible to work with him individually, it was clear that my supervising teacher was not. Usually a calm, gentle woman who was slow to lose her temper, seeing Matthew the student perform balancing acts worthy of Cirque du Soleil, and Matthew the student teacher turning a blind eye, would cause her to cry out: 'Matthew, what are you doing?!' I was never sure which one of us she had in mind.

At the end of my term I returned to the university to complete the theoretical component of my education degree, and was bemused by the contradictory approaches to behavioural problems presented to us by the Department of Education Psychology. Whereas some professors stated that the only worthwhile approach was to instil a rigid behavioural regimen of positive and negative reinforcement, others advocated a humanistic approach that was much more child-centred and still others favoured developmental and cognitive theories. A month later, returning to visit the classroom in which I had been teaching, I discovered that there was yet another approach. When I entered the room, the first thing I noticed was that Matthew had a different desk from all of the other students. They had replaced his two-piece desk, in which the chair and desk were separate, with one in which the chair was welded to the desk – no more circus routines for him. The second thing that struck me was that Matthew was still, sitting quietly at his desk and staring at a spot on the chalkboard. Unlike the other children, he did not seem to notice me, preferring, perhaps, to remain in his own little world. 'Matthew seems quiet today', I ventured to my supervising teacher. 'Yes,' she replied, 'he's been put on Ritalin. For his hyperactivity. He's much easier to handle these days.' I nodded, but was not sure that I liked what I saw. Sure, he was quiet, still, not bothering anyone. But where was his energy, his bounce, his vitality? Where was the kid that made me laugh in spite of myself? The kid who was so creative during art class and who excelled at gym? His behaviour was certainly less disruptive, but I wanted to see the other Matthew. I did not return to the classroom for any more visits.

It was not long before I encountered hyperactivity again. Feeling discouraged after my teacher training, I had opted for a job as a youth counsellor with the YMCA, helping teenagers who had dropped out of school. A large part of my job was helping these young people access government funding so that they could return to school. In navigating the complex funding structure, it soon became apparent to me and my colleagues that if a funding applicant was diagnosed with a disability, he/she not only had a much better chance of getting approved but also was given more leeway in terms of making academic progress. A disability diagnosis was a veritable get-out-of-jail-free card. Soon a good part of my day was devoted to spotting youth who might have such a disability, and hyperactivity was the disorder we most commonly identified.

For the most part, I saw little problem with this strategy. My job was to help troubled youth, kids who came from abusive backgrounds, had been involved in drugs, crime and gangs and who had often been homeless or in prison, to improve their lives. A hyperactivity diagnosis greased the wheels of bureaucracy; whether the kids we labelled were hyperactive or not mattered little to me if they got their lives back on track. Moreover, in identifying candidates for the diagnosis we were simply employing accepted criteria, and I genuinely trusted the mental health professionals who eventually, and inevitably, provided the official diagnoses and prescribed the pharmaceutical treatments. They, too, believed they were providing a lifeline to many of these troubled kids. I found the fact that I and most of my colleagues could also tick most of the diagnostic boxes ourselves quite amusing, but not overly troubling. There was the odd individual who made me wonder – like Larry, an eighteen-year-old who, despite his so-called disability, could manage six paper routes and wrote a 500-page manual for a role-playing game he created – but ultimately my concern was helping my clients, not questioning the system.

This all changed when I quit my job two years later to go back to university for an MA in history. My original proposal was to study the history of natural philosophy in England, specifically the impact of the Boyle Lectures on the relationship between science and religion. A perfectly good topic, I thought. But as I laboured through my Historiography of the History of Science course, wrestling with the likes of Karl Popper, Ludwik Fleck, Thomas Kuhn, Michel Foucault, Paul Feyerabend, Imre Lakatos, Bruno Latour and Harry Collins, I kept hearkening back to my experience at the YMCA and the notion of hyperactivity. Why had I never heard of hyperactivity growing up? Why had it become so ubiquitous? Why were we so quick to prescribe drugs, at the expense of cognitive and behavioural treatments, to treat hyperactivity? And why did we ignore the complex backgrounds of these young people in seeking an explanation for their behavioural, social and educational problems, preferring to explain away their problems in life on a genetic, neurological glitch? I decided that examining the history of hyperactivity was the best way to address such questions and, within three months of starting my degree, I abandoned Robert Boyle for Bart Simpson.

During the course of writing this book, I have been given another lens through which to interpret the behaviour of children. I am now the father of a very bouncy seven-month-old baby boy. To say that Dashiell is active is, well, what everyone says. He loves jumping in his Jolly Jumper, dancing vigorously with his dad and splashing gleefully in his bath. Although he seems to have good powers of concentration when a new object is presented to him, and he is already more dextrous than his father, it is altogether clear that he dislikes being still. Whereas most of the babies at the baby club his mother takes him to are content to stare quietly out of their prams, Dash insists on bouncing up and down on his mother's lap, attempting to make eye contact with everyone in the coffee shop. It is possible that at some point in the future someone will suggest that Dash is hyperactive. I hope I have the wherewithal at that point to refrain from commenting and instead suggest that they purchase this book.

So, what does this tell you about my approach to the history of hyperactivity? If anything, I hope it demonstrates that I do not come to the subject as an objective observer; I have seen hyperactivity from a number of different perspectives. I know as much as anyone that the concept of hyperactivity is complex and that decisive answers about the validity of the disorder and how best to treat it are elusive and often confounding. But that does not mean that it is impossible to reach a better, more sophisticated understanding of hyperactivity and how to approach the problem posed by troublesome children. It is possible, and the first step towards this improved understanding of hyperactivity is to come to grips with its history.

Introduction: Why the Hype?

Hyperactivity is all around us. If current estimates are to be believed, anywhere between 2 and 18 per cent of children in the United States, for example, have hyperactivity or Attention Deficit/Hyperactivity Disorder (ADHD). A recent survey of worldwide prevalence suggested that 5.29 per cent of the world's children had the disorder.[1] Most of us know a hyperactive child or, increasingly, an adult so-diagnosed, and even if we do not, we could probably describe one quite accurately. Hyperactive children tend not only to be overactive, but also inattentive, impulsive and often defiant and aggressive as well. They have difficulty at school, have problems in their relationships and may eventually struggle in the world of work. The disorder is also associated with higher rates of imprisonment, drug and alcohol abuse and other mental illnesses, particularly depression.

Popular representations of the hyperactive child, who tends to be a boy, also abound, and include Dennis the Menace, Calvin from the Calvin and Hobbes comic strip and, most notably, Bart Simpson. As young Bart discovers in a 1999 episode of *The Simpsons* entitled 'Brother's Little Helper', amphetamines, such as Ritalin (methylphenidate), are the most commonly prescribed treatment for hyperactivity, and have been so for half a century. Bart is tricked into taking a Ritalin-like drug called 'Focusyn' by his father Homer. Although he quickly becomes a model student, he also develops paranoia and starts behaving even more erratically than normal. By the end of the episode, his parents have switched him onto Ritalin, and the episode ends with Bart singing, to the tune of 'Popeye, the Sailor Man': 'When I can't stop my fiddlin', I just takes me Ritalin,

I'm poppin' and sailin', man!' Other television characters diagnosed with the disorder include junior member of the Soprano clan Anthony Jr. In a 1999 episode of *The Sopranos* entitled 'Down Neck', Anthony, Jr is diagnosed with hyperactivity by a school psychologist. Although his father Tony suspects that the disorder is nothing more than a 'way for these psychologists to line their pockets', and thinks that 'all he [Anthony, Jr] needs is a whack upside the head', his wife Carmela is appalled, demanding, 'You'd hit someone who's sick? You'd hit someone with polio?'

The dialogue between Tony and Carmela neatly highlights the divisive nature of hyperactivity. On one level, hyperactivity is an accepted psychiatric disorder. It has been included in the *Diagnostic and Statistical Manual of Mental Disorders* (DSM) in one form or another since 1968 and there is no doubt that DSM-V, expected in 2012, will also include another version of it. Although the aetiology of hyperactivity is sometimes described as complex or multicausal, most researchers believe fundamentally that it is an inherited condition that affects the executive functioning in the brain, possibly due to the imbalance of neurotransmitters. In part because of this widely acknowledged neurological explanation, the use of amphetamines is also approved in most medical circles, despite the fact that Ritalin has another life as a street drug and that it and other hyperactivity medication can cause alarming side effects, not to mention the dubious ethics of, and alarming precedents set by, giving children powerful drugs to control their behaviour. If sales of hyperactivity medication are considered, it is clear that most physicians, teachers and parents of hyperactive children believe that the risks posed by such drugs are far outweighed by the dangers posed by the disorder itself. In other words, hyperactivity is seen by the medical and educational establishment as a serious, neurologically based psychiatric condition that requires medical attention and pharmaceutical treatment.

Not everyone, however, accepts such views. Despite the official pronouncements about hyperactivity and its causes and treatments made by medical associations, such as the American Psychiatric Association, and lobby groups, such as CHADD (Children and Adults with Attention Deficit/Hyperactivity Disorder), hyperactivity remains a highly contentious topic in medical, education and parenting circles. The array of responses to a recent study linking hyperactivity and genetics provides an interesting example of how divisive the disorder can be. In September 2010, just as the new school year was getting under way, the following headline was splashed across the BBC website: 'New Study Claims "ADHD Has a Genetic Link"'. The study's author, Professor Anita Thapar of Cardiff University, was quoted as saying that the research, published in the Lancet, provided 'the first direct genetic link to ADHD', and argued that her findings should help reduce the stigma faced by the parents of hyperactive children who blamed themselves for their children's behavioural problems.[2] It did not take long for contrary opinions to emerge.

Oliver James, a clinical child psychologist and broadcaster, was asked by the BBC for his comments and subsequently rubbished the study, stating that the 'findings have been hyped in the most outrageous fashion', and contending that genes 'hardly explain at all why some kids have ADHD and not others'.[3] Fergus Walsh, the BBC's health correspondent, also cautioned that there 'is a danger of reading too much into [the] new research', adding that the 'bold claims do not seem to be borne out by the actual research paper'.[4] In the 245 comments appearing on Walsh's blog over the following days, the study, as well as James's critique, were either praised or reviled, with hyperactivity either described as an epiphanic explanation for intractable behavioural and learning problems or dismissed as an imaginary diagnosis and excuse for lazy and irresponsible behaviour. Doubters blamed increased rates of hyperactivity on everything from poor diet and bad parenting to not enough time spent in the outdoors and the devious marketing of profiteering drug companies. In contrast, the parents of hyperactive children condemned any suggestion that hyperactivity was not a legitimate medical problem, rooted in neurology and passed along in families. If anything was made clear by the 245 posts, it was that discussion of hyperactivity was bound to attract a wide range of diverse and impassioned perspectives, and precious little agreement or insight.

For anyone who has followed the debates about hyperactivity over the past half-century, the passion generated in such comments is not surprising. Ever since it began to be regularly diagnosed in North America during the late 1950s, and Ritalin was first used to treat it in the early 1960s, hyperactivity has been a controversial diagnosis. Two books published during the early 1970s illustrate how dichotomized opinions could be about hyperactivity's very legitimacy as a psychiatric disorder. In the first book, Camilla Anderson, who had served in California as the chief psychiatrist for the world's largest women's prison, believed that hyperactivity, which she called minimal brain damage, was a major factor in crime, drug abuse and welfare dependency.[5] The danger posed by hyperactivity was such that it warranted eugenic solutions, including the 'need for selective population control', 'changing age-old laws and values regarding abortion' and forced 'family limitation' through '"the pill", intrauterine devices (IUD), sterilization, or whatever techniques were reliable and nonmorbid'.[6]

On the other side of the debate were journalists Peter Schrag and Diane Divoky, who, in their provocatively titled book, *The Myth of the Hyperactive Child: And Other Means of Child Control*, argued that hyperactivity was not a valid medical disorder, but instead an example of coercive social control. According to them, the diagnosis was causing an entire generation of youth

> to distrust its own instincts, to regard its deviation from the narrowing standards of approved norms as sickness and to rely on the institutions of the state and on technology to define and engineer its 'health'.[7]

For Schrag and Divoky, who emphasized the role of pharmaceutical companies in popularizing the disorder, the tools used to identify, diagnose and treat hyperactivity 'all serve the purpose of legitimizing and enlarging the power of institutions over individuals'.[8] Depending on which book was read, hyperactivity could be seen as either an existential threat to the well-being of the state or a myth contrived to control children and benefit drug companies.

Although the views of Anderson and Schrag and Divoky may appear to be at the extreme ends of the spectrum, the hundreds of books written about hyperactivity since have also been characterized by polarized views, strong opinions and little compromise in attitudes or approaches. Some commentators, such as psychiatrist Peter Breggin, have claimed that the 'concept that "ADHD" is a biological or neurological disorder is entirely fabricated' and amounts to 'a cruel and unusual diagnosis'.[9] In complete contrast, others have suggested that such a diagnosis can be of enormous benefit to children and adults who 'have struggled all their lives, may have been diagnosed with other learning disabilities, or may now be plagued by a compromised self-image based on experiences of failure and frustration'.[10]

In other words, while some health professionals see hyper-activity as a specious, misleading and damaging label that harms, rather than helps, children, it is viewed by others as a source of salvation for struggling children and adults.

Experts who accept the existence of hyperactivity as a medical condition, however, do not always agree about what causes the dis-order. Although genetic, neurological theories remain prevalent, unconventional explanations for hyperactivity are common and span the spectrum of possibility. While some, such as Vancouver physician and columnist Gabor Maté, have suggested that hyper-activity has a strong developmental component rooted in early childhood experiences, others, most notably San Francisco allergist Ben Feingold, have argued that the disorder is triggered by food chemicals, particularly synthetic colours, flavours and preserva-tives.[11] Sugar, fluorescent lights, television, chemical cleaners, anti-biotics, pesticides and heavy metals, such as lead, as well as depleted levels of vitamins, minerals and fatty acids, have also been cited as environmental and dietary causes of hyperactivity, and lack of exercise and not enough time in the great outdoors have also been posited as possible explanations. Even chiropractors have had their say, suggesting that spinal misalignment is at fault.[12]

Many of the more socially based explanations for hyperactivity have also differed considerably from one another. On the one hand, psychologist Richard DeGrandpre believes that hyperactivity is a consequence of the United States' 'rapid-fire culture', which has 'created a nation hooked on speed and the stimulant drugs that simulate speed's mind-altering effects'.[13] On the other hand, psychoanalyst and broadcaster Thom Hartmann contends that hyperactive children and adults are hunters who have been left behind as humans left hunter-gatherer societies for civilizations based on agriculture. In other words, the genetic make-up of 'hunters', past and present, is imbued with the characteristics which would have been essential to people living as hunter-gatherers: traits such as constantly monitoring their surroundings (distractibility), being willing and able to take risks (impulsivity) and being capable of tireless pursuit of particular goals (hyperactivity).[14] In contrast, 'farmers' are more able to concentrate, exhibit patience and employ a cautious approach to life; such attributes serve such people well not only in agricultural settings, but also in the classroom and office. So, even if one was inclined to resist the conventional neurological explanations for hyperactivity, there are still plenty of theories from which to choose. Hyperactivity may be a neurological dysfunction, a hangover from our evolutionary past, a signifier of our increasingly chemicalized environment, the fruit of stressful family relationships or a symptom of a culture addicted to speed, unable to cope with real time.

On one level, many of these explanations make some sense. From one perspective, hyperactivity can be interpreted as a tool for social control just as easily as it can be seen as a genetic, neurological dysfunction from another. If we know that certain vitamin deficiencies, such as in the condition beriberi, can cause emotional disturbances, why would we doubt that other deficiencies, or exposures to other substances, might trigger hyperactivity? If we know that the first antipsychotic and antidepressant drugs were derived from coal-tar dyes, why is it so unfathomable that food dyes with a similar chemical ancestry can also affect behaviour? Similarly, it should not be too surprising to read that family distress can manifest itself in behavioural problems, just as it should not shock us that some of us are more or less disposed to have personal characteristics which are more or less helpful in different learning and vocational environments.

What is alarming, however, is that most hyperactivity theorists have been stubbornly unwilling to accept that hyperactivity is a complicated concept that can be justifiably interpreted in many different ways. Pluralism, it seems, is simply not part of their vocabulary. One reason for this is simple: pluralistic, relativistic explanations for controversial phenomena do not sell as many books as those that are polemical and singular. Another more important reason, however, is that most people who have commented and theorized about hyperactivity, in addition to most physicians who have treated the disorder, most parents and teachers of hyperactive children and most hyperactive children and adults themselves, know very little about its history. Moreover, what they do believe about its history is often inaccurate and misleading. In the wake of such ignorance, simplistic explanations, and treatments, abound. This book is an attempt to change that.

When the history of hyperactivity is examined in detail, a much more nuanced, compelling and instructive story surfaces, one that reveals insights into the complex ways in which culture, societal expectations, demography, professional politics, economics, ideology and patient activism create and continue to shape our understanding of what a mental illness is, and how to treat it. Some aspects of the story, much like the tale psychiatrist David Healy tells about the proliferation of depression as a common psychiatric condition, boil down to how medical professionals and pharmaceutical companies have, if not explicitly created, then aggressively marketed, new psychiatric conditions in order to promote particular intellectual ideologies and psychoactive products.[15]

It would be wrong, however, to argue that the emergence of hyperactivity has been solely a medical conspiracy. Concerns about hyperactive children, much like the worries about so-called feeble-minded children in late Victorian and Edwardian England that historian Mark Jackson has so aptly described, have also been rooted in national politics and fears about the intellectual fitness of the state and, particularly, its young people.[16] Likewise, it would be a mistake to assume that the popularization of hyperactivity has been the responsibility of powerful people, such as physicians, politicians and pharmaceutical executives, alone. Much like the construction and reconstruction of the concept of post-traumatic stress, as detailed by anthropologist Allan Young, the growth of hyperactivity as a medical and cultural concept has also been a grassroots phenomenon, shaped by patient lobby groups and disability rights associations.[17] Having said that, however, it is also true that the more one analyses how particular patients have experienced mental illness, the more varied such experiences prove to be. As with historian Ali Haggett's discoveries about the mental health of housewives in post-war Britain, individuals' specific understandings and experiences of hyperactivity have varied considerably, depending on how they have conceptualized the disorder, what it represents to them and how they have dealt with it.[18] Finally, before we judge too harshly the treatments, both conventional and unconventional, that have been afforded to hyperactive children, it is crucial to consider how and why such remedies have emerged. As historian Erika Dyck has shown in her fascinating study of the Saskatchewan LSD therapy experiments and Jack Pressman has demonstrated in his masterful exploration of psychosurgery, treatments for mental illness have needed to be politically, economically, ideologically and ethically acceptable, as much as they have been seen to be clinically effective.[19]

Put in more explicit terms, I argue that the only way in which to grasp the profound medical, cultural, educational and social implications of mental disorders such as hyperactivity and, in turn, resolve the often intractable debates that have hampered our ability to deal effectively with them, is to employ a historical approach. Specifically, if we are to comprehend why hyperactivity has become such a phenomenon and whether its emergence indicates fatal flaws in the ways in which we understand and treat mental illness, we must explore the wide range of social, cultural, economic, technological and political factors that have shaped our understanding of it during the past 50 years. There are, I believe, appreciable benefits in taking such an approach to the study of mental illness. For mental health professionals, the history of hyperactivity may indicate the need for more sophisticated, pluralistic and socially informed approaches to mental illness, and a reconsideration of the stifled ideologies that have resulted in simplistic, reductionist and inflexible thinking. It should also be a call to mental health professionals, and a reminder for health historians, to acknowledge how all medical knowledge is a complex construction, a conglomerate consisting of cultural, social, political, technological and scientific constituents that is forever changing, and not always for the better. For educators, hyperactivity's history raises questions not only about how we teach children, but also about the ultimate aims of education in a rapidly changing world. Finally, for parents of hyperactive children and those diagnosed themselves, this book is intended to do something different. In a society in which the meaning of health, particularly mental health, is increasingly altered without much of our own input, *Hyperactive* is meant to be an empowering story that can help people make more informed decisions about their own mental health and that of their children.

As a coda to this introduction, consider that I have been using the term hyperactivity to describe what is currently called ADHD or Attention Deficit/Hyperactivity Disorder. There are a number of reasons for this, but primarily the term hyperactivity is more historically consistent than the acronym ADHD, which only became prominent during the 1990s. It is also a term that most parents and physicians understand today and would have understood half a century ago. In other words, hyperactivity has been the term used most commonly and consistently to describe the children first diagnosed with hyperkinetic impulse disorder in 1957 and ADHD in 2012. Some, but not all, of the other terms used to describe what I call hyperactivity include hyperkinetic impulse disorder, organic brain syndrome, acting out, minimal brain damage, hyperkinetic reaction of childhood, minimal brain dysfunction, Attention Deficit Disorder (ADD) and finally ADHD.

These terms demonstrate the different ways in which hyperactivity has been perceived by the medical community since it emerged during the 1950s. In many ways, the first term employed to describe hyperactivity, hyperkinetic impulse disorder, was the most accurate in that it reflected that hyperactivity was not only a disorder of over-activity, but also one involving problems in impulse control. The psychiatrists who coined it worked at Emma Pendleton Bradley Home, a children's psychiatric institution in Rhode Island, and the technical-sounding term reflected the asylum's emphasis on biological psychiatry.[20] In contrast, acting out, a term often employed by psychoanalysts during the 1960s to describe hyperactive, impulsive children, denoted their belief that such behaviour was the outward expression of internal tensions, often rooted in domestic and social problems.[21] Other terms, such as minimal brain damage, a fairly generic term which was initially employed in the 1940s by Alfred Strauss and Heinz Werner and was later used to describe hyperactive children, delineated what many physicians believed to be at the root of hyperactivity, namely neurological trauma caused before, during or after birth. When it became apparent to clinicians that not all of their patients had a history of such trauma, the term was changed to minimal brain dysfunction, which similarly highlighted the neurological origins of hyperactivity, but gave no hint about the specific causes.

The term that became popular during the 1980s to describe hyperactivity, ADD, was also a conscious construction used to stress something particular about the disorder. First employed in DSM-III (1980) as Attention Deficit Disorder with or without Hyperactivity, or ADD, as it was called in both the medical and popular literature, the term centred on a completely different aspect of hyperactivity. Unlike hyperkinetic impulse disorder or hyperkinesis, which emphasized overactivity, Attention Deficit Disorder stressed inattention, which many researchers believed to be at the heart of the disorder. Placing the emphasis on inattention encouraged teachers and clinicians to be cognisant of not only children who were overactive and disruptive, but also those who were easily distracted, daydreaming their days away without causing any overt problems in the classroom. This change in terminology also meant that such professionals were increasingly on the lookout for ADD in girls, who were not diagnosed with the disorder to the same degree as boys. This gender inequality had bemused theorists who downplayed the social aspects of hyperactivity and wondered why boys were diagnosed over 2.5 times as often as girls.[22] By stressing inattention, not only were such discrepancies explained, but also many more children, and increasingly adults, became potential recipients of the ADD label and, subsequently, rates of hyperactivity escalated throughout the 1980s and 1990s.

By 1987, and the time that a revised version of DSM-III emerged, ADD had become Attention Deficit/Hyperactivity Disorder, or ADHD, placing hyperactivity once again at the heart of the disorder. Encapsulated in this infectious acronym were not only a wide range of behaviours that could be identified in millions of children and adults but also a sense of scientific legitimacy and gravitas that such acronyms often afford. More applicable than minimal brain damage or hyperkinesis, and less judgemental than acting out or minimal brain dysfunction, ADHD soon transcended the medical sphere and entered the vernacular to describe a certain type of child or adult whose difficulties adjusting to scholastic, vocational or social situations were no fault of their own or their parents, but rather due to a hidden neurological disability passed along in families and treated with drugs. Although hyperactivity had been recognized for 30 years, it was only after the term ADHD was coined that the disorder reached epidemic proportions and became not only a North American phenomenon, but also an international one. Of course such developments have not been entirely due to a name, but it is important to recognize the power of labels, particularly ones with which millions of people have been happy to be branded.

Calling this a history of ADHD, therefore, is somewhat misleading, partly for chronological reasons, but also because it conveys an inappropriate legitimacy to a concept that remains controversial and contested and that demands deconstruction. In other words, referring to hyperactivity as ADHD is to accept that hyperactive, inattentive and impulsive behaviour is, and always has been, pathological, of neurological and genetic origin, and warrants medical intervention. It also suggests that there is little in the social realm that can help us understand why such characteristics are deemed to be problematic, as a *New York Times* health columnist has recently argued.[23] As most medical historians would argue, nothing could be further from the truth. The history of hyperactivity is as much a story about changes in the political, cultural, technological, domestic and educational environment as it is a story about medicine.

ONE

Before Hyperactivity

If someone interested in hyperactivity looked at any one of the countless textbooks, self-help books, medical articles, newspaper stories and websites focusing on the subject they might think there was little need for a history of hyperactivity. This is not because the history of hyperactivity is uninteresting or serves little purpose, but rather because they might believe that this history has already been written. And to a certain extent, they would be correct. A version of the history of hyperactivity has been written and is often included in many such books and articles. While these histories are not identical, they do follow a similar pattern and all have the same purpose: to depict hyperactivity as a genetic and neurological condition that has been ever-present in humans and has little to do with the social environment.[1] For anyone familiar with the history of medicine, and psychiatry and mental health in particular, this should pose no surprise. History has often been employed not only to explain, but also to condemn or justify, current practices in medicine. There is nothing inherently wrong with this, but it should be incumbent upon the historian to ensure that the point being argued, whether it be critiquing the institutionalization of the mentally ill or rationalizing controversial practices such as lobotomy, does not get in the way of sound historical methodology. Unfortunately, this has not been the case in most textbook histories of hyperactivity.

The story such textbook histories tell proceeds as follows: The condition was first recognized in the mid-nineteenth century by German physician Heinrich Hoffmann, who in 1844 wrote a popular collection of nursery rhymes entitled *Der Struwwelpeter* (Shaggy

Peter in English). One of his creations was Fidgety Philip, who causes chaos at the dinner table. The tale then moves forward half a century and over to London. Here, paediatrician George Still made the first clinical observations of hyperactive behaviour in children, which he subsequently published in the Lancet. Although some accounts also mention the descriptions of one of Still's contemporaries, Thomas Clouston, most histories then fast-forward again, this time to the 1920s and the emergence of post-encephalitic disorder. Following the encephalitis epidemics of 1917 and 1918, physicians were confounded by a neurological condition that afflicted encephalitis survivors. Many of the symptoms, according to such histories, were similar to those found in hyperactivity. The history of hyperactivity then ends, apparently, in 1937 with the discovery made by Charles Bradley, at Emma Pendleton Bradley Home in Rhode Island, that amphetamines improved the school performance of his institutionalized patients. Bradley's use of amphetamines is seen to foreshadow the employment of other stimulants, particularly Ritalin, 25 years later.

And that, seemingly, is the history of hyperactivity. While some accounts, such as a chapter by prominent hyperactivity researcher Russell Barkley, provide more details and discuss scientific developments during the past 50 years, others, including the current Wikipedia entry for 'History of Attention-Deficit Hyperactivity Disorder' do not discuss anything after the 1917–18 encephalitis epidemic.[2] This does not mean that the search for hyperactivity in past centuries has ceased. Recently, for example, eighteenth-century Scottish physician, chemist and mineralogist Alexander Crichton has been heralded for providing an even earlier description of hyperactivity, which he called 'mental restlessness', a full century prior to Still's observations in the Lancet.[3] Many other physicians have engaged in retrospective diagnoses, claiming that figures such as Oliver Cromwell, Wolfgang Amadeus Mozart, Lord Byron and Winston Churchill were hyperactive cases. Such diagnoses not only help to explain away some of these luminaries' personal shortcomings, but also, for those who claim that hyperactivity has always existed, underline the longevity of the disorder, hinting as well that a hyperactivity diagnosis will not necessarily keep one out of the history books.[4] But why the disorder has become so prevalent in the past six decades, in contrast, is not something addressed in any textbook histories of hyperactivity.

There are two primary problems with the textbook approach. The first is that textbook histories focus on periods when hyperactivity, as a medical, educational and cultural entity, was simply unimportant, especially when compared to the more recent past. It might be possible to find very isolated cases in the medical literature prior to the 1950s where something like hyperactivity is described (although these must be analysed much more carefully as demonstrated below), but such examples are infinitesimally rare. Moreover, such cases are not discussed or echoed in the educational or popular literature, unlike during the last half-century. Cultural references to such children are also difficult to spot; the Bart Simpsons and Anthony Soprano Jrs are nowhere to be found. To put it crudely, such histories omit the best bits. It is akin to writing a history of Russo–American relations and failing to mention the Cold War. Or, to use a medical example, producing a history of HIV/AIDS without examining the toll it has taken in Africa. Scouring the distant past for evidence that hyperactivity has always been present is not inherently wrong, but it is misguided, particularly given how influential the disorder has become more recently and how much has been written about it.

The reason why the history of hyperactivity has been sought in past centuries and decades has been to reinforce the notion that such behaviour has nothing to do with the social environment; it is all about neurological factors which are rooted in genetics and, therefore, are timeless and universal. Competing explanations for such behaviour are conspicuously absent. For example, during the rare instances when hyperactivity was mentioned in medical journals prior to the 1950s, it was more often than not associated with allergies, especially food allergy. While Detroit paediatrician B. Raymond Hoobler described how food allergy could leave children restless, fretful, irritable and sleepless, T. Wood Clarke cited the 'case of a girl of ten years who was so overactive and unmanageable that, although she had an IQ of 139, she could not be handled at home and had to be sent to a special school' until her allergies were identified and treated.[5] The titles of many of these articles, including 'Puzzling "Nervous Storms" Due to Food Allergy', 'Allergy as a Causative Factor of Fatigue, Irritability, and Behavior Problems of Children' and 'The Relation of Allergy to Character Problems in Children', are as suggestive of hyperactivity as the writings cited in the textbook histories of hyperactivity, yet they are never mentioned.[6] It could be that the authors of such histories have never come across this literature, but it is also the case that allergic explanations for hyperactivity undermine the genetic, neurological theories that textbook histories of hyperactivity intend to support.

It is ironic that the children and behaviour described by food allergists are ignored, since they are much more reminiscent of hyperactivity than the observations that are cited in textbook histories. Indeed, the second problem with textbook histories of hyperactivity is that the examples they provide are simply not convincing. When the writings of Hoffmann, Clouston, Still and others are analysed it becomes clear that there are serious discrepancies between what they describe and what becomes known as hyperactivity much later. While it could be argued that the descriptions of such observers are what is at fault (in other words, the children that they witnessed were hyperactive, but not depicted in terms that we would understand), this seems to be an overly present-centred way of seeing the past. Historians should be loath to view the sources they analyse through a lens tinted by current ways of seeing the world. In order to demonstrate that the history of hyperactivity as we know it does not extend into the distant past in a meaningful way, and is instead a much more recent phenomenon, this chapter examines the six most commonly cited descriptions of so-called hyperactive behaviour. These include Alexander Crichton's description of 'mental restlessness'; Heinrich Hoffmann's mid-nineteenth-century nursery rhyme character, Fidgety Phil; the clinical observations of British physicians Thomas Clouston and Sir George Still at the turn of the twentieth century; the emergence of post-encephalitic disorder during the 1920s; and, finally, Charles Bradley's research during the mid-1930s on amphetamines and childhood behaviour. Analysis of these episodes demonstrates how, despite the fact that they have been cited repeatedly as being crucial moments in the history of hyperactivity, the childhood behaviours depicted by Hoffmann, Still and other physicians during the nineteenth and early twentieth centuries do little to support the claim that hyperactivity has long been of concern to physicians, educators and the general public. They also do nothing to address the question of why hyperactivity has become prevalent and so controversial in more recent decades, the answers to which would help us better understand the disorder today.

All of this is not to say that children and adults have only presented hyperactive behaviour during the last half-century. It is self-evident that some people, particularly children, have always been overactive, distractible and impulsive, and that these characteristics have presented problems to parents and teachers. But such characteristics have not always been seen as pathological, requiring medical attention and treatment with drugs, despite what textbook histories contend. As a recent article about Tom Sawyer and modern psychiatric conditions suggests, despite the fact that Tom

> clearly has Attention Deficit Hyperactivity Disorder . . . [he] turns out fine in the end. In 19th-century Missouri, there were still many opportunities for impulsive kids who were bored and fidgety in school. The very qualities that made him so tiresome – curiosity, hyperactivity, recklessness – are precisely the ones that get him the girl, win him the treasure, and make him a hero.[7]

In other words, behaviour that is deemed to be pathological in some contexts can be seen as positive in others. Therefore, in order to understand the emergence of disorders such as hyperactivity, it is essential to examine the contexts as much, if not more so, than the behaviours themselves. Textbook histories of hyperactivity do not do this; they fail to acknowledge that, as historian and neuropsychiatrist German Berrios has argued:

> the social criteria for selecting abnormal behaviours and the brain inscriptions identified for them do change with time.

This means that there is no transhistorical object of inquiry (i.e., an eternal mental disorder) which the psychiatry of today may expect to share with the disciplines that managed the 'phenomena of madness' before the nineteenth century or might share with disciplines that will be constructed to manage them.[8]

Instead, textbook histories of hyperactivity show how history can be exploited by interested parties to shape the understanding of a disorder, creating a more scientifically based history that, by ignoring the social, cultural and political aspects, accords with an acceptable version of how medical science operates.

Alexander Crichton and 'Mental Restlessness'

Despite the fact that most accounts of the history of hyperactivity cite George Still or Heinrich Hoffmann as providing the first descriptions of the disorder, an article by Erica Palmer and Stanley Finger contends that hyperactivity was described much earlier by Scottish physician Alexander Crichton (1763–1856).[9] Towards the end of Crichton's 1798 *Inquiry into the Nature and Origin of Mental Derangement*, he included a chapter entitled 'Attention and Its Diseases', which Palmer, Finger and others argue depicts hyperactivity.[10] Crichton described how

> the incapacity of attending with a necessary degree of constancy to any one object almost always arises from an unnatural or morbid sensibility of the nerves, by which means this faculty is incessantly withdrawn from one impression to another. It may be either born with a person, or it may be the effect of accidental diseases. When born with a person it becomes evident at a very early period of life, and has a very bad effect, inasmuch as it renders him incapable of attending with constancy to any one object of education.[11]

He proceeded to state that:

In this disease of attention, if it can with propriety be called so, every impression seems to agitate the person, and gives him or her an unnatural degree of mental restlessness. People walking up and down the room, a slight noise in the same, the moving a table, the shutting a door suddenly, a slight excess of heat or of cold all destroy constant attention in such patients, inasmuch as it is excited by every impression. . . . When people are affected in this manner, which they very frequently are, they have a very particular name for the state of their nerves, which is expressive enough of their feelings. They say they have the *fidgets*.[12]

What Crichton described does sound like hyperactivity, perhaps more so than any other entry in textbook histories of hyperactivity. His focus on attention, rather than overactivity, resembles especially how hyperactivity was conceptualized when the term Attention Deficit Disorder was introduced in 1980, emphasizing inattention for the first time. But there are also discrepancies between how Crichton viewed attention – and its diseases – and how it would come to be seen in the mid-twentieth century. These differences revolve around what compromises an individual's attention and how to improve the attention of those who struggle to focus. Crucially, Crichton focuses not so much on the individual and his/her deficiencies, but rather upon the environment and the many factors that impact upon attention. Coping with mental restlessness becomes as much about helping people recognize the educational and vocational circumstances in which they will thrive as it is simply improving their ability to concentrate.

Although physicians today acknowledge that there are differing degrees of hyperactivity, essentially the disorder is seen as a fixed medical condition. In other words, a child has hyperactivity or does not and if he/she does have it, he/she will have it for life. It is a label that, for good or ill, is constantly and forever attached to an individual and a lens through which his/her behaviour must be viewed. Crichton, in contrast, believed that attention was highly variable. Not only did attention vary naturally from person to person, but an individual's ability to concentrate also waxed and waned according to many factors. Particular circumstances, ranging from fatigue and disease to even a heavy meal, might affect one's concentration, and focus on one series of thoughts could either pass naturally to associated notions or be broken off by a more powerful stimulus, such as a flash of lightning, a sudden noise or physical pain.[13] The ability to withstand such distractions, according to Crichton, was also dependent upon volition or willpower, which also varied from person to person.[14] Here Crichton's discussion of attention was as much philosophical as it was medical in nature. The relationship between volition and attention, Crichton explained, was dependent upon whether or not one believes humans have free will, a philosophical matter. Philosophy, for Crichton, was tied inextricably to the issue of attention, something left unconsidered by today's hyperactivity experts, much to the detriment of our understanding of the disorder.

Unlike today's physicians, who prefer to treat hyperactivity with drugs, Crichton believed that an individual's powers of attention could be improved through better education. He bemoaned how many a child is 'kept for many years together to the irksome task of loading his memory with a vocabulary of mere words'.[15] Such children fell 'victim to mental fatigue, or else acquire a great disgust for instruction'.[16] But even more important for Crichton was acknowledging 'the great readiness with which we attend to certain subjects and objects rather than to others'.[17] It was clear to Crichton that

the peculiar idiosyncrasies, or dispositions of each individual, are seldom sufficiently attended to; and hence it frequently happens that many of our youth, although endowed with many natural talents, remain dunces during the early part of their lives. If they improve afterwards, it is owing to self tuition, or accidental circumstances having fortunately thrown such objects of science in their ways as are fitted to awaken new desires, and kindle the flame of curiosity in their minds.[18]

Crichton went on to argue that

every public teacher must have observed that there are many to whom the dryness and difficulties of Latin and Greek grammars are so disgusting that neither the terrors of the rod, nor the indulgence of kind intreaty can cause them to give their attention to them. If a boy of this disposition be found to be by no means deficient in natural understanding, why should many good years be lost in a fruitless attempt?[19]

Moreover, teachers should acknowledge that students had variable powers of attention and adjust their instruction accordingly. It is possible that such a child-centred educational philosophy might have been influenced by Rousseau's *Emile* (1762), in which the perils of ineffective instruction were delineated. Many men, according to Crichton, had they been

judiciously treated in their youth, might have become ornaments to their family, and useful members of society, but who having acquired an early disgust for study, have fallen a prey to false desires and wants, to the great prejudice of their health and fortune.[20]

Interestingly, Crichton observed that such inattentiveness was rarely seen in 'the lower classes of people', since their attention was 'sufficiently excited by their numerous wants, the pressures of which, by exciting acute desires, keeps the faculty alive'.[21] Social and educational circumstances, therefore, played a large role in determining one's power of attention.

Despite Crichton's emphasis on external factors, he also discussed how mental restlessness could result from nervous impairment. Although Crichton described how some people could be born with such a 'morbid sensibility of the nerves', he focused primarily on how other diseases, particularly those of the nervous system, but also febrile, respiratory and digestive diseases, could trigger such attentional impairments.[22] He also reassured his readers that when an individual was born with mental restlessness, 'it is seldom in so great a degree as totally to impede all instruction; and what is very fortunate, it is generally diminished with age'.[23] Finally, Crichton suggested that the best way to address such deficits was through student-centred educational practices.

Mental restlessness, therefore, was a highly complex issue for Crichton, one with educational, social, philosophical and medical aspects. Perhaps this complexity is one reason why hyperactivity expert Russell Barkley has remarked that Crichton's chapter is inferior to the articles written by George Still a century later (see below), in that it is less 'scientific' and 'scholarly'.[24] Leaving the question of what has passed for scientific and scholarly in different historical periods to one side, it is clear that Crichton's comments, particularly those dealing with education, complicate simplistic neurological descriptions of hyperactivity. When certain passages of his chapter are highlighted and taken out of context, it appears that Crichton did describe a disorder resembling hyperactivity. But when his chapter is read in its entirety, Crichton's analysis of mental restlessness and how to prevent it diverges considerably from the message of textbook histories of hyperactivity, providing a call to perceive attention and its diseases in a much more holistic, socially informed fashion. Perhaps it is not so surprising that Crichton's entry into textbook histories of hyperactivity has come so late.

The First Hyperactive Child?

Although Crichton discussed mental restlessness in students, the two case studies he described were of adults, not children, and, according to textbook histories, another half-century elapsed before the first so-called hyperactive child was described. This child did not emerge from a medical case study or an educational treatise, but instead in the form of a fictional character from a nursery rhyme. Fidgety Philip

> . . . won't sit still;
> He wriggles,
> And giggles,
> And then, I declare,

Swings backwards and forwards,
And tilts up his chair,
Just like any rocking horse –
'Philip I am getting cross!'

See the naughty, restless child
Growing still more rude and wild,
Till his chair falls over quite.
Philip screams with all his might,
Catches at the cloth, but then
That makes matters worse again.
Down upon the ground they fall,
Glasses, plates, knives, forks, and all.
How Mamma did fret and frown,
When she saw them tumbling down!
And Papa made such a face!
Philip is in sad disgrace.[25]

As mentioned above, Fidgety Philip was the creation of German physician, Heinrich Hoffmann (1809–1894), and was depicted in his children's book, *Struwwelpeter: Merry Stories and Funny Pictures* (published in German and English in the 1840s). Hoffmann's psychiatric work at a lunatic asylum in Frankfurt seems to have inspired those who cite Hoffmann's poem as the first identification of hyperactive behaviour. But Hoffmann's intent in writing *Struwwelpeter*, which includes nine other nursery rhymes, such as 'The Story of Little Suck-a-Thumb' and 'The Dreadful Story of Harriet and the Matches', was not to describe pathological child behaviour, let alone hyperactivity. Dissatisfied with the quality of children's literature, he wrote the poems to entertain his young son. As children's literature expert Jack Zipes describes: '*Struwwelpeter* is a funny manual of good sense . . . tell[ing] children, especially middle-class children, in graphic detail exactly what will happen to them if they do not do as they are told.'[26] In Hoffmann's words:

When the children have been good,
That is, be it understood,

Good at meal-times, good at play
Good all night and good all day –
They shall have the pretty things
Merry Christmas always brings.

Naughty, romping girls and boys
Tear their clothes and make a noise,
Spoil their pinafores and frocks,
And deserve no Christmas box.
Such as these shall never look
At this pretty Picture-book.[27]

Others have argued that Hoffmann's poems were not actually didactic, but instead a parody of such moralizing nursery rhymes. According to literary theorist Margaret R. Higonnet, Hoffmann drew the caricatures (which accompanied and preceded the poems) 'as a form of therapeutic communication intended to help his young patients overcome their fear of him'.[28] Rather than condemning, let alone pathologizing, such behaviour, Higonnet argues that 'Hoffman's medical experience and therapeutic experience strongly suggests that *Struwwelpeter* should be read . . . as a manners book which gives covert instruction in mischief'.[29] If this is so, then Fidgety Philip can be read as more of a celebration of rambunctious, exuberant behaviour, despite the messy consequences this might have for adults.[30]

Although Fidgety Philip avoids punishment for his behaviour, some of the other children are less fortunate. Harriet's dalliances with matches see her being burnt to a pile of ashes, Little Suck-a-Thumb ends up having his thumbs cut off by a rather draconian tailor and Cruel Frederick, who takes pleasure in hurting animals, suffers a topsy-turvy reversal of fortune. Nevertheless, nothing suggests that Hoffmann's characters were inspired by his clinical experiences. That most writers of textbook histories of hyperactivity have not examined *Struwwelpeter* in detail, let alone in context, is further evidenced by another one of Hoffmann's characters, namely, 'The Story of Johnny Head-in-Air'. Johnny's inattentiveness, which sees him tumble into a river when distracted by acrobatic swallows, could be seen as being an example of a child with an attention deficit as easily as Fidgety Philip's naughty, restless behaviour can be perceived as representing hyperactivity.

When physicians have looked at Hoffmann's stories in more depth, however, they have mistakenly interpreted the attributes of his mid-nineteenth-century characters from twenty-first-century perspectives, engaging in unhelpful present-centred history. Psychiatrists J. Thome and K. A. Jacobs, for example, have analysed *Struwwelpeter* and connected nearly all the behaviours exhibited with late twentieth-century pathologies, ranging from what they describe as 'dissocial racist behavior' to eating disorder.[31] With respect to Fidgety Philip, Thome and Jacobs argue that Hoffmann 'had noted all of the details which today would lead to a clear diagnosis'.[32] This claim is problematic not only because a single episode of misbehaviour would not justify a 'clear diagnosis' for most psychiatrists, but also because it presupposes that such behaviours have always been seen as pathological. Children have long played with matches, sucked their thumbs, hurt animals and ruined dinner, but this does not mean that such behaviours have always been perceived in terms of mental disorder. Instead of medicalizing the behaviours exhibited by fictitious nursery-rhyme characters from the mid-nineteenth century, perhaps more effort should be made to examine why similar behaviours have been avidly pathologized during the last 50 years.

Fin de Siècle Descriptions of Pathological Children

There are very different reasons to distinguish the behaviours depicted in the next section of the textbook history of hyperactivity from modern notions of the disorder. Most such accounts cite the speech of Sir George Still (1868–1941) to the Royal College of Physicians of London in 1902 as the first mention of behaviours resembling hyperactivity in a medical context. Psychiatrists Seija Sandberg and Joanne Barton, however, have referenced earlier observations of disruptive children, especially those made by Thomas Clouston (1840–1915) in 1899.[33] Clouston, a lecturer at the University of Edinburgh and Physician Superintendent of the Royal Edinburgh Asylum, described three 'very difficult morbid conditions in neurotic children, conditions which lie on the borderland of psychiatry', specifically, 'simple hyper-excitability', 'hypersensitiveness' and 'mental explosiveness'.[34] As with the omission of 'Johnny Head-in- Air', it is strange that Clouston is rarely mentioned in textbook histories of hyperactivity because his descriptions of these conditions are superficially more similar to today's depictions of hyperactivity. Clouston's portrayal of the hyper-excitable child who 'becomes ceaselessly active, but ever-changing in its activity' and suffers from 'undue brain reactiveness to mental and emotional stimuli' neatly encapsulated the hyperactivity, impulsivity and distractibility that have typified hyperactive children for the last half-century.[35]

Important differences also existed, however, between the children Clouston described and the hyperactive children who emerged during the mid-twentieth century. First, he stated that hyperexcitable behaviour 'only lasts for perhaps a few months or a year', which differed from later claims that hyperactivity was more permanent, lasting until puberty, if not forever.[36] Second, he emphasized that mentally explosive children, who were prone to irritable, impulsive, violent and defiant behaviour, were most often girls, not boys. This contrasts with later descriptions of the epidemiology of hyperactivity, which demonstrate that rates of the disorder are higher in boys. Many psychiatrists believe that girls have been under-diagnosed because they tend not to exhibit the 'explosive' behaviour that Clouston associated with his female patients. Instead, girls diagnosed with ADHD are thought to be calm, but inattentive and unable to focus.[37] Nevertheless, Clouston's observations, not to mention his preference for using 'large doses' of bromides to treat such children, 'to the point when the symptoms of brominism [mental dullness, loss of coordination and, sometimes, skin eruptions] are beginning to show themselves', and his belief that such conditions were rooted in the cerebral cortex, bear greater resemblance to today's understanding of hyperactivity than those that followed during the next 50 years, including the often-cited observations of George Still.[38]

Still is best known generally for being one of Britain's first paediatricians and for describing Still's Disease, a form of juvenile arthritis. For hyperactivity experts, however, his fame comes from describing 'children who show a temporary or permanent defect in moral control . . . but pass for children of normal intellect' and were not otherwise believed to be insane.[39] Such children are acknowledged by many physicians, and some historians, to be the first hyperactive children described in the medical literature.[40] Still believed that such defects in moral control were pathological, not simply variations on normal childhood behaviour, and that they could be caused by a number of factors. He was also bemused by the fact that while brain injury or illness could trigger such defects in some children, others presented no history of such neurological trauma.

Still's definition of 'moral control' was similarly expansive, encompassing 'the control of action in conformity with the idea of the good of all [and] . . . the good of self'.[41] These defects resulted in a wide range of behaviours including, in order of frequency, 'passionateness [susceptibility to passion, intensity of emotion or anger]', 'spitefulness-cruelty', 'jealousy', 'lawlessness', 'dishonesty', 'wanton mischievousness-destructiveness', 'shamelessness-immodesty', 'sexual immorality' and 'viciousness'.[42] At the heart of these characteristics was 'the immediate gratification of self without regard either to the good of others or to the larger and more remote good of self'.[43]

When the twenty cases Still presented are analysed, however, they appear far removed from the children diagnosed with hyperactivity later in the twentieth century. First, Still stated that he had to make a 'special effort to seek out' the twenty children that made up his study; such cases were 'by no means common'.[44] This is not surprising when the histories of the children he described are examined. Still's patients appear to be significantly disturbed, capable of inflicting brutal violence on other children, their parents, animals and themselves, and many were either institutionalized or thought to be headed for such a fate.

Most of the specific behaviours Still described were also either distinct from or not necessarily associated with hyperactivity today, including pica (eating inedible substances such as dirt or paper), extreme violence, self-harm, pathological dishonesty, sexual

immorality and theft. Inattention and fidgety behaviour were mentioned, but they were not the core symptoms that Still illustrated.
In the case of Still, as well as that of Clouston to a lesser extent,
hyperactivity was only one of a series of symptoms of underlying
pathology; it was not a disorder in itself. What Still and Clouston did
accomplish was to identify a small group of children who were neither intellectually disabled nor brain damaged, but whose troubling
behaviour was similar to children with such conditions. In so doing,
they began the process of applying medical terminology and aetiology to socially and educationally inappropriate behaviours exhibited
by children. It is more this process, rather than the identification of
hyperactivity in children, which bears a resemblance to the research
conducted by child psychiatrists on hyperactivity half a century later.

Still's descriptions of defective moral control, as well as
Clouston's observations, also highlight how perceptions of childhood behaviour were tied to political and cultural trends. Still's
emphasis on defects of moral control reflected late Victorian concerns about behavioural and intellectual disability in children and,
especially, children who were not so impaired that they would be
routinely placed in an asylum. As historian Mark Jackson has
described, individuals who occupied 'the borderland of imbecility'
were believed to be a burden on society and a potential threat to
social order.[45] Both the children Still described and those diagnosed
with hyperactivity decades later occupied such a borderland, a conceptual space, as Jackson puts it, 'ambiguously situated between the
supposedly pathological and the normal'.[46] The desire to categor-
ize such individuals 'appears to have been inspired not primarily
by cognitive developments in science and medicine but by the
administrative, educational, and medical problems generated by
institutional expansion in the middle decades of the nineteenth
century'.[47] The education legislation during the 1860s and 1870s
which required that more children attend school, and exposed those
who had difficulty learning, also contributed to the interest in and
classification of marginal learners. As we will see in the next
chapters, similar pressures on the education system, as well as
changes to the provision of psychiatric care, also affected the
debates about hyperactivity during the 1960s.

It is also important to consider Still's own character and motives in assessing his observations. Recall that Still depicted the behaviours he witnessed as 'defects in moral control'; indeed Still's stance on issues of morality might well have influenced his views on childhood behaviour. Still was a lifelong bachelor who never had his own children, spending his spare time reading classical literature in the original Greek, Latin, Hebrew and Arabic instead. He was described by a contemporary as 'a model of propriety', 'reserved', 'rigidly Victorian', 'conservative by nature'; 'he never told a funny story; he never wanted to hear one'. Given the first chair in paediatrics in England, he was also '"abnormally reticent" except with small children [especially girls, whom he preferred to boys] between the ages of three and ten'.[48] While this description should not raise suspicions about the veracity of Still's observations, it might make one consider how Still might judge childhood behaviour and assess its morality. Although mere speculation, it could be that Still idealized young children, and especially girls, seeing them as particularly innocent and precious. Perhaps when their behaviour strayed from what he saw as normal, becoming passionate, spiteful and shameful, he interpreted this as being pathological when others might perceive it as variations of what was normally expected in children. Again, such comments are speculative, but they do raise the importance of context in assessing historical descriptions of behavioural phenomena. Context, as the following chapters suggest, is key in understanding any aspect of hyperactivity and its history.

Post-encephalitic Disorder

Context is also important in the next instance of hyperactive behaviour commonly cited in the textbook histories, namely, that found in people suffering from post-encephalitic disorder during the early 1920s. Encephalitis lethargica, von Economo disease or sleeping sickness, was a perplexing disorder that grew to epidemic proportions during the late 1910s, only to disappear during the late 1920s. While the disease resulted in a wide range of symptoms, including lethargy, fever, headache and catatonia, its residual effects, described as post-encephalitic disorder, were equally troubling and included physical impairments, eating disorders, sleeping abnormalities and socially disruptive behaviour ranging from 'excessive naughtiness to gross criminal acts'.[49] For instance, Franklin G. Ebaugh, director of the Neuropsychiatric Department at Philadelphia General Hospital, stated that sexual precocity was exhibited in two of the seventeen cases he saw, and that violent behaviour was evident in many others. While one 'patient tried to kill other members of his family', another 'stabbed a schoolmate with a knife'.[50] Ebaugh also cited depression (including suicide attempts), hysteria, involuntary tics, insomnia, narcolepsy, dizziness, headaches, visual disturbance and mental deficiency as other common symptoms.[51] The prognosis of post-encephalitic disorder was thought to be severe enough in some cases to warrant leucotomy (lobotomy), although this practice also needs to be put into its historical context.[52] In two reported cases the adult patients, who had contracted encephalitis when they were children, were 'content and happy', yet 'still irresponsible . . . as judged by normal social standards', following their prefrontal leucotomies.[53] The wide range of symptoms included in post-encephalitic disorder was even more diverse than those described by Still, but the cause of the disorder echoed Still's description of 'morbid defect of moral control associated with physical disease'.[54] Whereas Still associated such behaviour with diseases and injuries ranging from tumours and meningitis to blows to the head and acute rheumatism, the cause of post-encephalitic disorder was made clear by its name: the symptoms were only present following encephalitis.

This association of abnormal behaviour with neurological trauma, resulting from infection, injury, auto-immune dysfunction or pre-natal or post-natal respiratory problems explains why post-encephalitic disorder has had a place in textbook histories of hyperactivity, despite its symptoms being so much more severe. The episode would encourage subsequent researchers, including Eugen Kahn and Louis Cohen during the 1930s, and Alfred Strauss and Heinz Werner during the 1940s, to study in more depth the link between brain damage and behavioural problems.[55] While the former pair's term 'organic drivenness' is often suggested as a precursor to hyperactivity, the latter pair described what they called 'minimal brain damage', a term that would also be associated with hyperactivity until it was replaced by the less aetiologically specific 'minimal brain dysfunction'.

Such associations were important in the history of child psychiatry in that they helped to establish for many professionals that such disturbing behaviour was rooted in neurological, rather than psychological, dysfunction. In the words of a Dr Myerson, who commented on Kahn and Cohen's presentation to the Massachusetts Psychiatric Association in 1933:

> I think that encephalitis has probably illuminated the genesis of personality more than all the psychological work that has been done. I say this with all due respect to the psychologists who are here present.[56]

In other words, childhood behaviour disorders were diseases of the brain and not the mind. Similarly, to the writers of textbook history, post-encephalitic disorder cements into place the notion that hyperactivity has little or nothing to do with environmental factors, such as domestic experiences, education, social conditions or nutrition, and everything to do with neurology. As with the rest of the textbook approach, it simplifies and medicalizes what is a much more complicated and multifaceted phenomenon.

Amphetamines and Hyperactivity

The final episode listed in textbook histories of hyperactivity had implications for how the disorder would come to be commonly treated. At Emma Pendleton Bradley Home, the children's psychiatric asylum in Rhode Island mentioned above, the prevailing belief during the 1930s was that psychiatric problems were largely neurological in nature, and that neurosurgical remedies were often warranted.[57] This reflected the beliefs of many American psychiatrists during the 1930s; the psychoanalysts from Nazi Germany and elsewhere in central Europe, who would come to dominate post-war American psychiatry, had only just started their exodus to North America. Charles Bradley (1902–1979), a great nephew of the Bradley Home's

founders, headed the medical staff and utilized pneumoencephalo-
graphy in his neurological evaluation of patients. The painful
procedure involved draining much of the cerebrospinal fluid from
around the brain with a spinal tap and replacing it with oxygen,
helium or air in order to improve X-ray images of the brain.[58]

This was the procedure the possessed child Regan MacNeil
(whose behaviour does seem to resemble one of Still's children)
endured in the 1973 horror film The Exorcist. By the 1980s, computed
tomography (CT) scans had largely replaced the painful and dangerous procedure, but during the 1930s the operation resulted in
severe headaches and nausea. Bradley prescribed the amphetamine
Benzedrine to his patients in an effort to stimulate the replacement
of spinal fluid and relieve the children's headaches. The drug did
little for the headaches, but teachers at Bradley Home observed that
it seemed to improve the ability of patients to learn and behave at
school.[59] After testing the drug further, Bradley began using it
regularly, and published his observations in the American Journal of
Psychiatry. By 1950 he had used it on 275 children and found that it
was effective over 60 per cent of the time.

Although the American Journal of Psychiatry has described
Bradley's discovery as one of 'the most important psychiatric treatment discoveries', they also recognized that while

> Bradley and his colleagues published their observations in
> prominent journals and they were reported in the media as
> well, 25 years passed before anyone attempted to replicate
> his observations, and more than 25 years passed before
> stimulants became widely used for ADHD.[60]

Why was this the case? In some ways, drugging children would
seem to be a relatively tame intervention during the 1930s. This was
the era when other types of neurologically based psychiatric
treatment were emerging, including insulin shock therapy (1933),
electroconvulsive therapy (1934) and leucotomy (1935). Given the
invasive and dangerous nature of these treatments, it is difficult to
imagine that psychiatrists would be averse to prescribing a stimulant, even to children.

The problem with Bradley's discovery had less to do with the supply or acceptability of the treatment than the demand for it. Bradley stumbled onto his findings trying to ease the headaches of children who had undergone a spinal tap; his observations that Benzedrine appeared to improve learning and behaviour were merely tangential. If there had been a greater demand for treatment alternatives for hyperactive children during the late 1930s, it is likely that Bradley's article in the *American Journal of Psychiatry* would have had more of a sudden impact. The fact that it did not do so suggests that such children were not perceived to be of major psychiatric concern until much later, when Bradley's discovery was taken up with alacrity. Most textbook histories, however, gloss over this 25-year gap and emphasize the long tradition of using stimulants to treat hyperactivity. Bradley's discovery might have provided a reference point to which later child psychiatrists could refer in order to stress the legitimacy of using stimulants to treat hyperactivity, but there was no established tradition of prescribing stimulants to children with behaviour problems until the emergence of drugs such as Ritalin during the 1960s.

It is likewise difficult to connect investigations of children's behavioural disorders during the early part of the twentieth century to conceptions of hyperactivity which emerged during the late 1950s. First, hyperactivity and inattention were only two of a wide range of behavioural problems identified by Clouston and Still and listed as symptoms of post-encephalitic disorder and minimal brain damage. They were also not as readily apparent or striking as other behaviours exhibited in these conditions, such as the extreme violence, criminal behaviour and self-harm also described. Children exhibiting such symptoms were also a rarity, due to the relative infrequency of childhood diseases and injuries that could inflict such damage on the brain.

Furthermore, unlike the vast majority of cases of hyperactivity that would be diagnosed during the 1960s, the cause of post-encephalitic disorder and minimal brain damage was self-evident. Since brain injury was not evident in the histories of most patients, researchers investigating hyperactivity during the 1960s and onwards could only speculate about aetiology. Because of this, by the 1960s researchers had largely replaced 'minimal brain damage' with the vaguer term 'minimal brain dysfunction', which could include both brain-damaged individuals and those whose neurological dysfunction was of unknown origin.

The clinical circumstances surrounding hyperactive children described during the first part of the twentieth century were also different from those of hyperactive children in later decades. Most early articles which mention hyperactivity concentrated on behaviours exhibited by children suffering from readily identified conditions, such as brain injuries, infections or allergies, rather than children whose hyperactive behaviour was unexplained. Others, including Charles Bradley's much-cited observations on the effect of stimulants on learning, were written about children whose previous psychiatric problems were such that they were already confined to psychiatric institutions. In these cases, hyperactivity was a symptom associated with particular, pre-identified medical conditions, rather than a behaviour believed to be pathological on its own. This is one of the key distinctions between the handful of articles written about hyperactive behaviour prior to the 1950s and the thousands of articles published since.

If the links between the descriptions of Crichton, Hoffmann, Still and others and how hyperactivity was depicted during the late 1950s are so tenuous, then why are they emphasized in most accounts of the disorder's history? One reason is that such histories fit into the traditional way in which medical history has been described, particularly by physicians. As sociologist Adam Rafalovich describes, medical accounts of the history of hyperactivity have discussed 'the history of ADHD as one characterizing the progress of modern clinical practice, slowly honing its nomenclature to greater levels of scientific validity and practical effectiveness'.[61] Hyperactivity, according to such accounts, fits into the broader notion that modern medicine is a progressive, ever-improving enterprise. Moreover, by extending the history of hyperactivity into past centuries, the notion that the disorder has always existed in the human population as a genetic, neurological glitch is reinforced. In this way hyperactivity is reified, transformed from a contested, controversial and socially constructed hypothesis into an eternal and universal biological fact. If we accept such accounts of the history of hyperactivity without question, then we are also likely to forget about the other side of the equation: the circumstances in which such behaviour is seen as problematic. And this is the subject that is addressed next.

TWO

The First Hyperactive Children

On 12 March 1951, Hank Ketcham first published the American version of 'Dennis the Menace' – in a bizarre twist of fate, the un-related British Dennis first hit the pages of the *Beano* five days later. When physicians and educators want to describe the characteristics of a hyperactive boy, they often mention Dennis the Menace as a per-sonification of the disorder. So, is it appropriate to describe the American Dennis as a hyperactive child? If the content of the comic strip is used as a guide, then the answer is no. Created a number of years before hyperactivity became a distinct childhood disorder, Dennis does get into trouble an awful lot and has an unfortunate tendency to irritate his parents and long-suffering neighbour Mr Wilson. But when Dennis is described, positive words are employed; words such as precocious, enthusiastic and energetic are used, rather than impulsive, distractible and hyperactive. Dennis is not depicted as having a mental disorder; instead, he is portrayed as a normal American five-and-a-half-year-old, definitely more active and less inhibited than his friends, the pensive Joey and the super-cilious Margaret, but certainly not to a pathological extent.

The fact that Dennis the Menace has been co-opted by hyper-activity experts as one of the many poster boys of the disorder demonstrates that something changed between when he was created and when his characteristics began to be perceived in a more negative fashion. When did boys like Dennis begin to be seen as hyperactive? If Dennis was not the first hyperactive child, who was? A quick foray into any medical search engine suggests that one possible answer to the first question is 1957. This was the year in which the first of a great wave of medical papers about hyperactivity was published, a wave that has not ebbed since.[1] As for who the first hyperactive child was, it is impossible to say, but it is safe to assume that he was an American, male and, given that he was diagnosed during the late 1950s, he was a member of the Baby Boom generation. Why was this the case?

The answer to this considerably more difficult question is central to any meaningful understanding of why hyperactivity has become such a pervasive phenomenon during the last 50 years. It is also the sort of question that many historians have asked with respect to the proliferation of other mental disorders during the same period. Depression, post-traumatic stress disorder (PTSD), anorexia nervosa, generalized anxiety disorder (GAD), obsessive-compulsive disorder (OCD) and oppositional defiant disorder (ODD) are just a few of the mental disorders that have either emerged in the last half-century or have morphed from being obscure conditions to becoming commonplace. As with hyperactivity, it is possible to find textbook 'histories' of these disorders that emphasize how they have always existed, providing retrospective diagnoses as proof. And, likewise, when the histories of these disorders are analysed in depth, the question quickly shifts from 'did such conditions exist in the distant past, thus justifying their legitimacy?' to the more pertinent, 'why have they become so prevalent now?'

For psychiatrist and historian David Healy, rates of mild and moderate depression mushroomed in conjunction with the development of drugs that could treat such disorders in the 1950s. Pharmaceutical companies did not only market their antidepressants and tranquillizers aggressively, they also sold the idea of mild and moderate depression itself. Although countless societal factors, ranging from decreasing stigmatization of depression to the existential angst of an increasingly secular society, have also been influential, a quick look at how pharmaceutical companies advertised the ubiquity of depression in medical journals beginning in the 1950s does lend credibility to Healy's argument.[2]

In other cases, the emergence of post-war mental disorders has had grassroots elements. Anthropologist Allan Young's research, for example, discusses how the traumatic experiences of Vietnam War veterans contributed to the establishment of PTSD as a valid condition. Although Young acknowledges that the notion of traumatic memory emerged in the nineteenth century, there are clear differences from how psychiatrists such as Sigmund Freud and Pierre Janet conceptualized the notion, as well as the idea of shell shock that is associated with the First World War, and what was described as PTSD in DSM-III.[3] Rather than being timeless, PTSD is

> glued together by the practices, technologies, and narratives with which it is diagnosed, studied, treated, and represented and by the various interests, institutions, and moral arguments that mobilized these efforts and resources.[4]

Likewise, Young argues that the concept of traumatic memory changes over time in accordance with societal preoccupations.[5] Just as the memory of the Vietnam War was beginning to fade, the destruction of the twin towers on 11 September 2001 traumatized a new generation of Americans. Not only were New Yorkers directly affected by the terrorist attacks seen to be at risk of PTSD, people from other cities, and particularly children, were also seen to be susceptible due to extensive television coverage of the event.[6]

The history of hyperactivity bears some resemblance to both that of depression and PTSD. As with depression, drug companies marketed the notion of hyperactivity as much as their ability to treat it. Hyperactivity, similarly to PTSD, has also been promoted by lay people, particularly parents whose children have struggled academically, as well as adults who see a hyperactivity diagnosis as an explanation for their vocational, educational and social difficulties. Lobby groups, such as CHADD, have also played a considerable role in marketing the notion that hyperactivity is a real, disabling and treatable neurological condition. And as with depression, PTSD and other mental disorders, there are many other reasons for the emergence and proliferation of hyperactivity. The answers to why hyperactivity has become such a ubiquitous medical phenomenon are many and they are complicated. The following chapter touches on many of these factors, but also highlights two of them in particular. The first has to do with the label itself, and how it could be applied to so many American children. The second involves why the label was applied with such enthusiasm during the late 1950s.

What's in a Label?

Labels are important in any discussion of mental illness. As described above, hyperactivity has been given many labels, each emphasizing different aspects of the disorder, its aetiology, prognosis and treatment. Similarly, changes in the labels used to describe other mental illnesses have also encapsulated significant changes in how those conditions have been understood. Transitions in terminology, for instance, from dementia praecox to schizophrenia, from multiple personality disorder to dissociative identity disorder and from shell shock to PTSD, to name but a few, reflect not only changes in medical thought, but have also affected who might be diagnosed with such disorders.[7] The shift from the term manic depression to bipolar disorder during the past few decades, according to Healy, reflected paradigmatic shifts in terms of how psychiatrists classified, explained and treated such a disorder.[8] Compared to the term manic depression, which emphasized the depressive aspects of the disorder, bipolar disorder indicated that the other side of the spectrum was equally important in determining diagnosis. The term bipolar also caught on in popular culture and became somewhat fashionable, being associated with creative people, such as musicians and artists, and mercurial personalities from both history and contemporary culture.[9] Members of the bipolar fraternity include comedian Russell Brand, children's author Robert Munsch, musician Sinéad O'Connor and actor Stephen Fry, who hosted a BBC documentary on the subject in 2006. Finally, 'a mania for pediatric bipolar disorder' emerged, resulting in a good deal of controversy surrounding why the disorder was being diagnosed in children and treated with mood stabilizers.[10] Of course, many other factors contributed to the boom in bipolar diagnoses in the 1990s and 2000s, not least of which, according to Healy, was the role of pharmaceutical companies in 'disease mongering', but the shift in terminology, and what that terminology implied, was also vital.[11]

The minting of a readily applicable label was also essential to the popularization of hyperactivity. In 1957, child psychiatrists Maurice Laufer and Eric Denhoff, along with Gerald Solomons in one paper, published two articles on 'hyperkinetic impulse disorder'. On the surface, there was nothing unusual about their research. They had all worked at Bradley Home under Charles Bradley and conducted their research on residents being treated there for 'psychoses, neuroses and behavior disorders'.[12] Unsurprisingly, they cited Bradley as an influence, but did not mention any other supposed hyperactivity pioneers, such as Clouston, Still, Kahn or Strauss. As with Bradley, they recommended the use of stimulants for hyperactive patients and employed electroencephalogram (EEG) images to explore the brains of their patients.[13] What was remarkable about the disorder they described, however, was how easy it was to apply to an astoundingly wide range of American children.

There were three reasons for its applicability. First, and most importantly, Laufer and Denhoff restricted their attention to a narrower range of behaviours than their predecessors.[14] Unlike Still and post-encephalitic disorder researchers, who were concerned chiefly about violent and immoral behaviour, the Rhode Island psychiatrists were interested in characteristics which would affect the schoolwork of children and were the first psychiatrists to link hyperactivity to academic performance. Although they listed 'hyperactivity; short attention span and poor powers of concentration; irritability; impulsiveness; variability [of behaviour and school performance]; and poor school work' as characteristic of such children, they stressed that 'hyperactivity is the most striking item'.[15] The name they chose also reflected this emphasis and, while their precise terminology did not endure, the disorder they described did. As paediatrician Howard Fischer noted recently in the *Journal of Pediatrics*, there are only minor differences between Laufer and his colleagues' conception, description and understanding of hyperkinetic impulse disorder in 1957 and what is believed about hyperactivity or ADHD today.[16] The label enabled subsequent researchers and clinicians to focus on a specific, yet easily applicable, constellation of behaviours which they could then identify, diagnose and treat.

The second aspect of hyperkinetic impulse disorder which Laufer and Denhoff stressed was its ubiquity. Despite the fact that their studies concentrated on institutionalized children, they emphasized that hyperkinetic impulse disorder was 'very common'. Indeed, among the 50 children they sampled from Bradley Home's population, 32 'presented the symptom picture of hyperkinetic impulse disorder'.[17] Furthermore, the authors implied that the difference between children with such a diagnosis and their undiagnosed companions might be difficult to determine:

> One striking point is that the characteristics which have been described are to some extent normally found in the course of development of children. That is, as compared with adults, children are hyperkinetic, have short attention span and poor powers of concentration, and are impulsive . . . In the course of their development, they outgrow this mode of behavior and actually, in the course of time, so do most of the children with the hyperkinetic syndrome.[18]

The hyperkinetic children Laufer and his colleagues described, therefore, had far more in common with 'normal' children than did the decidedly disturbed and violent children described by Still and those researching post-encephalitic disorder. Although they did not discuss epidemiology specifically, Laufer and Denhoff did stress that hyperkinetic children were usually of 'normal intelligence' and described how the disorder would be present in children attending mainstream schools, thus indicating that the disorder would not be restricted to institutionalized children, such as those living at Bradley Home.[19] In so doing, they also emphasized how such a disorder would contribute to educational problems and that its treatment would improve academic achievement. Accordingly, hyperactivity became an educational, as well as a behavioural, disorder.

Finally, Laufer and Denhoff unwittingly returned to one of Still's conundrums, which had not been applicable to researchers studying post-encephalitic disorder and minimal brain damage. Specifically, if obvious neurological damage from trauma or infection was only causing some of the behavioural problems they observed, what was causing it in the other cases?[20] Of the 32 children in Laufer and Denhoff's sample, only eleven (34 per cent) 'had a clear-cut history of commonly accepted factors capable of causing brain damage, such as head injury, encephalitis or meningitis early in life'.[21] In other words, a little over a third of these children could be described as having minimal brain damage or Strauss syndrome. The authors postulated that neonatal difficulties and 'purely emotional cause[s] might help to explain the aetiology of hyperkinetic impulse disorder', but emphasized that their thoughts on the subject were merely speculative.[22]

Unlike the conditions typically cited in the textbook history of hyperactivity, the disorder that Laufer and Denhoff described had the potential to become a widespread phenomenon. Although it was made up of a smaller range of symptoms than Still's defect of moral control or post-encephalitic disorder, such behavioural characteristics were more common and were seen in fairly normal children, rather than only in brain-damaged children. Operating within a predominantly psychoanalytic psychiatric paradigm, the authors also integrated psychoanalytic terminology, theory and treatment (psychotherapy) into their exposition of hyperkinetic impulse disorder, thus making the disorder acceptable and treatable for both biological psychiatrists and psychoanalysts. Unlike the previous incarnations of hyperactivity cited in medical texts, hyperkinetic impulse disorder could be applied not just to a small number of severely disturbed children, but also to a large percentage of the child population. The 1957 papers of Laufer and Denhoff provided a point of departure for modern conceptions of hyperactivity by depicting the disorder as one that could be applied to millions of children. It did not take long for dozens and then hundreds of researchers to begin studying hyperactivity, and by 1968, when the disorder was included in DSM-II, it was recognized as a disorder of epidemic proportions in the United States.

There were other reasons for the label's applicability. As child psychiatrist Justin M. Call suggested two decades later, the 'label of hyperactivity owes its popularity to the soothing effect such simple conceptions have upon issues of great cognitive complexity'.[23] In other words, hyperkinetic impulse disorder presented teachers, physicians and parents with a facile way in which to perceive what was a highly complex and inextricably multifaceted issue, namely how to explain why children misbehaved and under-performed in school. 'He's hyperactive', quickly became a catch-all explanation for problematic behaviour. Although one might doubt the validity of the term and question those who used it so readily, by the 1960s, most people certainly knew what it meant.

In this way, hyperkinetic impulse disorder can also be construed as what historian of science Ilana Löwy has called a 'loose concept', a notion containing elements of fluidity and indeterminacy. In Löwy's case, the concept of 'self' (or biological individuality) in immunology was loose enough to have 'facilitated interactions between scientists and physicians belonging to distinct scientific traditions'.[24] Löwy proceeds to state that 'imprecise concepts may help to link professional domains and to create alliances between professional groups'. This appears to be the case in the history of hyperactivity as physicians representing a number of disciplines (for example, paediatrics, psychiatry, neurology and general practice) were able to interact successfully with psychologists, educators, social workers and even parents to legitimize the concept of hyperactivity and validate the means by which to treat it.[25] Or as contemporary educator James McCarthy described: 'the confluence of state legislation, parental demand, federal funds, and professional concern has created an urgent demand that the education needs of such children be met'.[26]

As much as hyperkinetic impulse disorder had the potential to become applicable to millions of children, however, much more must be involved in the genesis of a new psychiatric disorder; sweeping categories and novel labels do not automatically attract patients as moths to a flame. So what were the circumstances that catapulted hyperactivity into medical and cultural prominence? What happened between the publication of Leo Kanner's seminal textbook Child Psychiatry (1957), which lacked any mention of hyperactivity, and the mid-1960s, when the 'mere mention of the term "hyperkinetic syndrome" is guaranteed to stir up vigorous discussion in medical, psychological, social work, and educational circles'?[27] Why did the disorder first emerge in the US? Although many of the profound changes to American society during the 1950s and 1960s played a role in the origins of hyperactivity, the prime catalyst had much to do with the Cold War and another event associated with 1957: the Soviet launch of two *Sputnik* satellites.

Post-*Sputnik* Panic

There are good reasons why rates of mental illness in general were seen to increase during the post-war period. During the Second World War, two million individuals were rejected for service by the American military for psychiatric reasons, raising the spectre that mental illness was rife in the American population.[28] While this realization gave a boost to the American psychiatric profession, particularly psychoanalysts, it also demonstrated how the exigencies of war could shape not only the economy, politics and science, but also transform ideas about what personal and behavioural characteristics young Americans had to embody in order to become productive citizens. Such expectations only increased during the Cold War, as the rivalry between the US and the Soviet Union spread from Third World battlegrounds to the Olympics, outer space and the classroom, infiltrating countless aspects of American life as a result. Crucially, the children born during the years following the Second World War, the Baby Boom generation, were seen to play a considerable role in the struggle with the Soviet Union for ideological and educational superiority.

It was in this political climate, marinated in the gloom of the Cold War and the threat of nuclear annihilation, that hyperactivity emerged. As the Soviet Union developed hydrogen bombs and launched the first satellites and humans into space, many influential Americans grew convinced that the US was losing the 'brain race', and unless the scholastic performance of all American children improved markedly, they would lose the Cold War altogether. This persistent perception contributed to the growth of hyperactivity diagnoses in three ways. First, as American politicians, educators and scientists began analysing why they were falling behind the Soviets, they came to identify and subsequently demonize the behaviours seen to interfere with high educational achievement.

The behaviours associated with hyperactivity, neatly encapsulated in hyperkinetic impulse disorder, were quickly recognized as being particularly damaging to learning and targeted by educators.

Second, critics of American education became concerned not only about the scholastic achievement of the intellectually gifted, but also about those believed to have average or even below average intelligence. The combination of Cold War competition and the increasingly automated workplaces created a demand for workers who could cope with elevated levels of technological sophistication, meaning that all children were expected to attain higher education standards. As Palmer Hoyt, publisher of the *Denver Post*, argued, 'the Russian corps of skilled technological brains now totals 2,700,000', and the US needed to revamp its education system in order to catch up.[29] This meant that all children, including academic under-achievers, were expected to stay in school longer than previous generations and achieve higher standards for graduation. In these circumstances, young adults who would have previously left school for work, where the behaviours associated with hyperactivity were not necessarily detrimental, were now expected to stay in school where they were seen to be problematic.

The final way in which *Sputnik* and the Cold War contributed to the emergence of hyperactivity involves the creation of a new educational profession, the school counsellor. School counsellors worked with teachers to identify hyperactive children who were struggling academically, label their deficiencies and refer them to physicians for diagnosis and treatment. Through this function, counsellors served as the lynchpin between the educational and medical spheres in the diagnosing of hyperactivity, ensuring that what was initially an educational problem became a medical issue as well.

In this way, the hyperactive child became symbolic of perceived American intellectual inferiority and the target of politicians, physicians and educators who saw improvement in academic achievement as essential to American security. The link between national defence and the emergence of educational pathologies is not unprecedented. The Cold War roots of hyperactivity mirror the development of novel notions of mental deficiency in Britain during the years before and after the Boer War. As Mark Jackson has demonstrated, concerns about the intellectual fitness of young Britons, which were intensified during the Boer War, spurred educators and physicians to identify individuals who were believed to be mentally deficient but not to the extent of idiots or imbeciles. These 'feeble-minded' individuals, occupying 'the borderland of imbecility', were thought to be the cause of numerous social 'evils', and an even 'greater danger to the State, than the absolutely idiotic', partly because they were less identifiable.[30] As Jackson contends: 'the borderland of imbecility was increasingly construed as a discrete, pathological entity, displacing the "urban residuum" of working-class slum dwellers as a major threat to social health'.[31] Similarly, concerns about American educational achievement during the Cold War contributed to a shift in the types of behaviour and sorts of students seen to be troublesome and in need of educational and medical intervention.

Much like feeblemindedness, hyperactivity was fabricated in response to political tension and occupied a borderland between 'the educationally and socially normal and the pathological'.[32] But before exploring the link between the Cold War and hyperactivity more closely, it is important to consider some of the other factors impacting upon the education system in the years following the Second World War. During this period, American schools were suffering from stresses emanating from a multitude of sources.[33] Chief among these was the emergence of the Baby Boom generation, the 75 million children who were born between 1946 and 1964.[34] Ironically, the women who gave birth to this generation, the largest cohort in American history, were members of the smallest cohort born during the twentieth century, specifically, those born during the 1930s. The Baby Boomers overloaded a school system that was already suffering from infrastructure deficits incurred during the Great Depression and the Second World War. Schools were also coping with teacher shortages, as many female teachers, in accordance with general trends among women during the late 1940s and 1950s, stayed out of the profession or left to marry and bear children at a young age.[35] As contemporary education commentator Paul L. Gardner described:

in these days of crowded classrooms, expanding enrol-
ments, and the rapidly changing world in the complex
society of today, teachers across the land are hard pressed to
deal adequately with their responsibilities for the welfare of
their students.[36]

Other educators commented that 'serious shortages in trained
teachers, classrooms, and up-to-date equipment, accentuated by a
marked bulge in school age children', were all contributing to a
'crisis in education'.[37]

Researchers, including those interested in hyperactivity, also
acknowledged that a direct link existed between overcrowding
and behavioural and academic problems. None other than Laufer,
Denhoff and Solomons asserted that overcrowding could cause
difficulties for children who had a tendency towards hyperactivity
and distraction, as well as their beleaguered teachers:

in the crowded classrooms of today, the teacher often
becomes hostile to the child who, despite seemingly good intelligence, can not sit still, can not keep his mind on his work,
hardly ever finishes the assigned task and yet unpredictably
may turn in a perfect paper. . . . The child frequently fails to
gain a proper foundation for the fundamentals of schooling
so that each successive year he falls progressively behind.[38]

Although the authors assumed that hyperactivity was a pre-existing
condition which was exacerbated by the crowded classroom, as well
as the hostility of the overworked teacher, it could also be argued
that the reverse was more accurate. In other words, children taught
by a stressed teacher in a teeming classroom were more likely to be
perceived as troublesome, and to be singled out for being so.

The impact of the Baby Boom generation on the school system,
however, was not simply due to the numbers of children entering
the school system. Historians Steven Mintz and Susan Kellogg argue
that American society during this period was 'filiarchal' – that is,
dominated by and greatly concerned with American children.[39]
From buying a house in the burgeoning suburbs because it was

believed to be a safer place to raise a family and a juvenile products industry worth over 30 billion dollars per year to the birth of television and rock and roll, much of American life centred on the economic, social and cultural interests of youth. Filiarchy, however, was not always seen by all to be a positive development. Franklin Ebaugh, who had researched post-encephalitic disorder during the 1920s, cautioned against 'child-centered' American culture and urged that the whims of children not overshadow the needs of society. In his view, over-indulgence created 'no more than a permanent "child," a psychological cripple perennially seeking meanings on the prairies of Beatnikville, instead of fulfilling his future in Communityville'.[40] In other words, children had to be educated to serve society, rather than their own egocentric desires.

Such thinking was compounded enormously in 1957 when the Soviet Union launched two *Sputnik* satellites into orbit. That the supposedly backward Soviets were the first into space was a shock to the American military, scientific and educational establishment.[41] The impact of *Sputnik* on the psyche of American educators and politicians was neatly illustrated in the following poem by Steven A. Modée:

Post-Sputnik Panic

when the bears
hurled a spaceball
into heaven
from left field
us got real scared
us expanded our spaceball program
us expanded our vocabulary too
us expanded everything
'till us then got the man in the moon
hah!
us beat them bears
yep!
us showed them bears
a giant leapfrog for all mankind[42]

Modée's poem captured not only the fear that Sputnik instilled in Americans, but also the sense of academic inferiority which accompanied the launch of the satellite. Accordingly, many conservative educators and politicians, such as Hyman Rickover (1900–1986), James Conant (1893–1978) and Max Rafferty (1917–1982) identified the education system as the scapegoat for American intellectual shortcomings. According to authors Barbara Ehrenreich and Deirdre English:

> Sputnik hit like a spitball in the eyes of American child-raising experts, educators and Cold War propagandists . . . Communist children were co-operative and good-tempered to a degree that was almost eerie compared to the Dennis-the-Menace personality deemed acceptable in American kids.[43]

Contemporary educators felt such critiques acutely, complaining that 'the Soviet firing of Sputnik into space seemed to unloose a veritable Pandora's box of criticisms of us'.[44] To many, Sputnik made 'American public education . . . the object of vigorous and widespread criticism and attack without parallel in our history', placing 'our schools . . . under terrific fire'.[45] According to prominent child psychologist, Erik Erikson, 'a sense of crisis has been aggravated by the long cold war and the sudden revelation of the technological strength of a supposedly "backward" rival'.[46]

One of the critics' primary targets was the progressive education movement, envisioned by philosopher John Dewey (1859–1952) and characterized by democratic, experimental, egalitarian and, above all, child-centred learning. Education historian Diane Ravitch has contended that by the 1940s progressive education was 'the dominant American pedagogy, . . . the conventional wisdom, the lingua franca of American educators'.[47] In theory, progressive education sought to provide children with practical, tangible experiences in which they would learn skills and knowledge to prepare them to be productive members of American society. According to one of the movement's proponents, Columbia professor William Heard Kilpatrick (1871–1965), the progressive approach would equip 'the child to face his future by learning to face intelligently his immediate present'.[48] They might, for example, learn about biology, arithmetic and economics by growing vegetables on school property and then selling them at a market to teachers and parents. In such active circumstances it was possible that many children with hyperactive tendencies would go unnoticed, if not thrive.

Creating such environments, however, was not easy and placed considerable burdens on educators. Dewey, who was not the most accessible of writers, was often misunderstood, particularly with respect to how rigorous he thought such classrooms should be, despite their child-centred nature.[49] The progressive classroom might look chaotic and aimless, but beneath the surface countless learning experiences were in place. Similarly to the educational philosophy described in Jean-Jacques Rousseau's *Emile*, pupils seemingly learned through accidents that were actually carefully planned. Accordingly, teachers in progressive classrooms had to be highly skilled and educated in order to ensure that such experimental projects resulted in learning and not chaos. As a *March of Time* newsreel of the late 1940s described, teachers were the 'keystone of Progressive Education . . . Necessary qualifications: ingenuity, patience, a thousand eyes, great physical endurance!'[50]

Despite these high expectations, many progressive classrooms were thought to be disordered and rudderless, failing to teach children the most basic of academic skills. As a father in the same newsreel asserted: 'Now, hold on Miss Fox. It's all very well to teach my boy to paint pretty pictures and build birdhouses, but he doesn't even know his multiplication tables.'[51] Although progressive education was on the wane by the 1950s, it continued to exorcize conservative educators and politicians, serving as a symbol for them of what was wrong in American education. *Sputnik* demonstrated to critics of progressive education that a return to more strict, subject-centred, authoritarian and structured classrooms was not only pedagogically more effective, but also vital to national security. The promise of progressive educators to provide schools that were 'actually fun' seemed frivolous to their critics in the midst of the space race and they, along with other child experts, including Benjamin Spock (1903–1998), bore the brunt of blame for American academic shortcomings.[52]

Indeed, fear that 'the Soviets have gone far ahead of us in the production of trained minds in science and technology', precipitated scathing critiques of American education from educators, scientists, politicians and military men.[53] Some of the most notable attacks on American education included Admiral Hyman Rickover's *Education and Freedom* (1959), James Conant's *The American High School Today* (1959), Arthur S. Trace's *What Ivan Knows That Johnny Doesn't* (1961) and Max Rafferty's *Suffer, Little Children* (1962). Admiral Rickover, well known as the 'Father of the Nuclear Navy', contended that 'the schools are letting us down at a time when the nation is in great peril. To be undereducated in this trigger-happy world is to invite catastrophe.'[54] Educator Asa S. Knowles (1909–1990) echoed these sentiments, warning that

> this sphere [Sputnik] tells not of the desirability but of the URGENT NECESSITY of the highest quality and expanded dimensions of the educational effort . . . the future of the twentieth century lies in the hands of those who have placed education and its Siamese twin, research, in the position of first priority.[55]

Physicist Lloyd Berkner (1905–1967) was equally convinced that 'brainpower [was] the resource upon which our nation must depend for its future economic and social health'.[56] Although most of the critics focused on science, others, such as English professor Arthur S. Trace, argued that the US also lagged behind the Soviets in the study of the humanities.[57] Whereas young Soviet children were likely to read Tolstoy, their American counterparts were only expected to contend with Dick, Jane and Spot the dog.[58]

The message in such publications was clear: education was to be the battleground on which the Cold War would be won or lost and, as of 1957, the dominant view was that the Soviets were winning. For most critics the solution to this perceived catastrophe was to reject the 'fun and games' approach of child-centred progressive education, which had dominated pedagogic philosophy since the 1930s, and to institute a more rigid, academic and standardized system in which firm, federally established objectives would be set out for students to achieve.[59] Substantial efforts would be made to identify struggling students' barriers, address them through various remedial measures and encourage them to stay in school and reach their academic potential.[60] Such recommendations were largely, though not universally, endorsed by educational administrators and found support in two pieces of federal legislation, most notably the National Defense Education Act (1958), but also the Elementary and Secondary Education Act (1965).[61]

The National Defense Education Act (NDEA), seen by its creators and observers as a direct reaction to Sputnik, invested one billion dollars to improve the teaching of science, mathematics, English and foreign languages at all levels of schooling, to hire guidance counsellors and to prevent students from dropping out of school. To Arthur S. Flemming (1905–1996), the Secretary of Health, Education and Welfare when NDEA was signed, the Act signified 'that education is a national unifying force' and demonstrated that 'an educated citizenry is the country's most precious resource'.[62] Sputnik might have been 'a blow to American pride', but for Flemming it also 'awakened and spurred us into rigorous self-examination of the total education system'.[63] The Soviet satellite, therefore, was seen by many as a blessing in disguise.

Even by virtue of its name, NDEA highlighted the link between educational achievement and military power. War, during the first atomic decades, was seen as a scientific enterprise, privileging brains over brawn. The relative strength of the superpowers was judged by how many nuclear weapons each side possessed, how powerful they were and how quickly they could be called into action. Flesh and blood soldiers almost seemed irrelevant. Space, similarly, was perceived chiefly in terms of what it implied about one's military power, rather than being seen as a worthy scientific enterprise in and of itself.[64] To a large degree, these assumptions were proved false by subsequent events. The Vietnam War proved catastrophically to Americans that, regardless of how many nuclear, not to mention chemical and biological, weapons they possessed, the predominant mode of conflict of the late twentieth century was guerrilla warfare, requiring and costing thousands of soldiers. Similarly, the exploits of the Apollo 11 lunar mission in the summer of 1969 indicates that many of the goals of NDEA were realized, but then the space programme foundered, as the political expediency of the space race faded away. But one crucial educational legacy remained; as expectations of American students increased, the characteristics of children unable to excel academically were thrust under the spotlight.

Future Scientists and Underachievers

As the educational achievements of young Baby Boomers were increasingly scrutinized, hyperactivity, impulsivity and inattentiveness became associated with academic underachievement and, by extension, the intellectual shortcomings of young Americans. Such traits, conglomerated in hyperkinetic impulse disorder, were thought to be particularly damaging in the educational fervour of the late 1950s because they were thought to prevent otherwise intelligent children from achieving educational success. An example of such associations is illustrated in a study published in the periodical *Exceptional Children* in the early 1960s which reflected the perceived failures in the educational system. The authors recognized that there was 'great concern about the use of talent in our society' and wanted to find ways to address the 'wastage in the [educational] system'.[65] Their task was to compare impulsivity rates in 'underachievers' with those of 'future scientists' who had been accepted into a summer space camp. The authors found that the 'future scientists' were not only much less impulsive than their underachieving classmates, but also more able to control their motor activity or, in other words, less hyperactive.[66] The study's conclusion was that the impulsive, hyperactive behaviour displayed by the underachieving students was the key distinction between them and the 'future scientists' desired by critics such as Conant and Rickover. Other contemporary researchers also stressed the importance of impulse control in academic success, and that controlling one's impulses was largely an innate activity. As one educator described, 'the ultimate and highest goal in so-called control comes not from the teacher or group domination, but with the establishment of self-control within the individual'.[67]

Concern about impulsivity and hyperactivity echoed a shift with respect to which behavioural characteristics were deemed to be most pernicious by American educators, physicians and politicians. Whereas shy, withdrawn and neurotic children who tended to be inactive were of greatest concern prior to the late 1950s, the increased premium on intellectual achievement following the launch of Sputnik meant that the most acute apprehension swung to excessively active children.[68] As child psychiatrist Gregory Rochlin noted, commenting on the previous trend:

> motor activity in the young child, even if excessive, is more favourably regarded than its opposite. Although the child who is hyperactive may be as emotionally disturbed as the shy inhibited child, the latter is apt to receive more attention than the former.[69]

Or, as educator Alice Keliher described the situation, mental health workers 'are more troubled about withdrawing, shy, really sick children'.[70]

By the late 1950s, however, educators become more concerned with overly active, rambunctious children, rather than those who were inactive, introverted and reclusive. This shift is reflected in Katherine Reeves's 'The Children We Teach' series in Grade Teacher, which changed its focus from shy, withdrawn children to children like ten-year-old 'Charles', who presented many of the symptoms of hyperactivity. Charles had

> quick dark eyes, restless hands and body and unreliable co-ordination which seems to come because he cannot synchronize his ideas and his movements. He slips from one interest to another, intense in his preoccupation of the moment, absorbing the essence of each, but moving insatiably from one activity to the next. Speed, movement, rapid-fire questioning, impatience, and irritability when he cannot manipulate situations successfully are characteristic of his behaviour.[71]

The title of Reeves's article, 'Each in His Own Good Time', suggested that she advocated patience in dealing with such children, certainly more patience than many of the education critics would have liked. Indeed, she hoped that Charles would be able to work with greater concentration, yet retaining his intensity and his 'essential personality'.[72] But, given the pressure that Sputnik had placed on the education system, the symptoms associated with hyperactivity were increasingly treated seriously as a problem of significant educational and medical importance.

Changes in child development theory during the 1960s also contributed to the notion that children like Charles had to be identified, diagnosed and treated, rather than gently guided through their development, as Reeves might have preferred. Specifically, paediatricians and child psychiatrists were beginning to question developmental theorists such as Erik Erikson, who thought that many of the pathologies of childhood and adolescence were social in origin and transitional in nature. Instead, many psychiatrists began to fear that disorders such as hyperactivity would persist into adulthood and hinder the individual's employability and work performance, perhaps becoming as debilitating as chronic depression and schizophrenia.[73] According to James F. Masterson, Erikson's dangerous ideas prevented a therapeutic intervention, an intervention that could be a crucial encounter for the adolescent.[74] Educators also recognized that the 'cost of prevention is far less than the cost of breakdown and its treatment' and that they, too, were involved in identifying problems such as hyperactivity and impulsivity.[75] Hyperactivity in schoolchildren, therefore, became seen as a precursor of not only academic underachievement, but also subsequent mental health problems that could cost the state in countless ways.

There were also subtler ways, however, in which hyperactivity became emblematic of academic underachievement. A series of Kellogg's breakfast cereal advertisements in Grade Teacher, for instance, featured a trio of troublesome children, all of whom displayed different symptoms of hyperactivity. 'Window-watchin' Wendy', who 'skips class right in her seat' represented the inattentive child; hyperactive children were characterized by the 'restless and irritable' 'Lemon-drop Kid'; and the 'Clockwork Kid', who was liable to be the 'mainspring of a classroom rebellion', embodied the impulsive, defiant child.[76] According to Kellogg's, however, these children did not need a revamped educational system but a better breakfast, ideally one found in a Kellogg's Corn Flakes box.

That a company such as Kellogg's had picked up on the concern about inattentive, hyperactive and impulsive schoolchildren indicates how problematic such behaviours were thought to be by the late 1950s. Such children have always caused trouble for parents and teachers, as characters like Fidgety Philip suggest. But following Sputnik, hyperactive children were increasingly singled out as both educationally and psychiatrically troublesome, instead of the withdrawn, shy children who had previously caused concern. The 'eggheads', who were previously dismissed as weak and inferior, were now seen with new respect, as numerous educators observed.[77] Or as Viscount Hailsham declared in a speech to the Royal Society in late 1957:

> A country neglects its eggheads at its peril. . . . It is the egghead who invents the Sputnik, not the captain of football, or the winner of the sword of honour . . . It is the egghead who discovers penicillin, who splits the atom, who thinks of the printed circuit, the electronic brain, the guided missile in the world of science.[78]

In the fervour for cultivating such eggheads, educators, parents and politicians were increasingly disturbed by children such as Reeves's 'Charles' and found that disorders like hyperactivity provided a suitable explanation for why they struggled to succeed.

No Place in Society for the Dropout

During the first half of the twentieth century, it would have been likely for 'Charles', as well as 'Window-watching Wendy', the 'Lemon-drop Kid' and the 'Clockwork Kid' to have left school in their early teens for vocations that would have suited their various personalities and aptitudes. Following the launch of Sputnik, however, the opinion of many education critics was that this was no longer acceptable; there was 'no place in society for the dropout'.[79] Instead, a sizeable improvement in high school completion rates were thought to be a necessary condition of the competitive, technologically sophisticated workforce that could once more out-perform the Soviets in scientific development. In the words of Stafford L. Warren, who served as an adviser to Presidents Kennedy and Johnson in the area of mental retardation, the US could 'no longer ignore the early school dropout on the excuse that we need a large labour force of uneducated muscle men'.[80] As President Johnson himself stressed: 'jobs filled by high school graduates rose by 40 per cent in the last ten years. Jobs for those with less school-ing decreased by nearly ten per cent'.[81] Dropping out of school to find unskilled work, therefore, a choice made then and now by many hyperactive students, was no longer considered an option.[82] Al-though the proportional rates of early school leavers were actually falling, and had been falling for half a century, the perception was that school dropouts were not only a national problem, but a matter of 'national security'.[83]

Sputnik was not the only factor contributing to the perception that more young people had to finish high school and ideally go on to college. Americans were also concerned about the increasingly automated workplace and the disappearance of unskilled work. According to United States Labor Department estimates, by 1970 only 5 per cent of jobs would be of the unskilled variety.[84] Also im-portant was the Servicemen's Readjustment Act of 1944 (commonly known as the GI Bill), which gave returning servicemen funding to complete higher education. The GI Bill's success was such that in 1947 returning servicemen accounted for nearly half of all college admissions and by 1956, the final year of the original bill, nearly half of the sixteen million American Second World War veterans had attended an educational programme.[85] This not only meant that college education was afforded to working class veterans who might not have otherwise had the opportunity, it also meant that the children of such veterans were also expected to graduate high school and attend college.

But for those concerned about matching the achievements of the Soviets, high school graduation alone would not win the 'brain race'. In order to train more scientists, engineers and technicians, critics such as Rickover not only demanded more graduates, but also desired higher standards for high school diplomas, including more hours of classes, more homework and attainment of higher levels of education in a shorter amount of time.[86] James Conant, the former president of Harvard University and ambassador to West Germany, believed that higher standards should be attained especially in core subjects, such as English, mathematics, foreign languages and science.[87] For Conant, these expectations applied not only to middle-class students in the burgeoning suburbs, but also to poorer students in the slums of the American cities.[88]

Although the higher standards were supposed to contribute to an increasingly technologically sophisticated workforce, there were drawbacks to such an approach. According to research presented to the American Psychopathological Association in the late 1960s:

as a result of increasing emphasis on academic credentials as prerequisite to occupational success, years of schooling have been continuously prolonged ... current pathways of vocational development are encumbered with hurdles that make the transition to work seem more like an obstacle course than a choice of desirable alternatives.[89]

High standards could also serve to discourage students, as a letter to the editor of *Science* indicated:

after Sputnik, the educators suddenly became infected with the idea that the day of reasonable [homework] assignments was over; from then on, students had to complete at least 100 problems per assignment in addition to increased reading assignments. Each instructor seemed to take the attitude that his assignments should occupy all of a student's waking hours.[90]

The author of the letter argued that such an 'overwhelming amount of homework reduced the student's ability to really learn his subjects' and resulted in students becoming 'disenchanted with science and engineering', the opposite effect of what Conant and Rickover had intended.

The higher standards also put the shortcomings of under-achievers under the microscope. As *New York Times* education columnist Dorothy Barclay explained:

> The school picture . . . in 1958, reflected almost entirely a tightening-up. But in some classrooms or communities, unfortunately, it was more like a cracking down. Concern about college admissions and general anxiety about America's technical ability, as highlighted by the space race, combined to produce demands for higher standards of achievement in the upper elementary grades and in high schools. The switch has given new incentive to some young-sters, but, where misapplied, its sudden severity has put a strain on others who have been unable, through lack of adequate preparation, to meet the new demands. . . . Even more significant to the average family, however, is the amount of attention being given to smoking out and stimulating the efforts of the under-achievers. These youngsters of varying abilities who are not working up to their potential.[91]

Writing in 1959, two years prior to when Ritalin was first marketed to children, Barclay was probably not aware of the irony inherent in her phrase 'smoking out and stimulating the efforts of the under-achievers'. Nevertheless, Barclay did recognize that higher educa-tional standards highlighted the academic difficulties of those students who, in previous decades, would have left school for employment in their early to mid-teens. Such students, whose penchant for being active and energetic was viewed as positive in many labour-intensive careers, were now expected to stay still in their seats and attend to lectures. Indeed, researchers recognized that hyperactive, inattentive children showed 'extremely poor advancement' with respect to the 'increasing emphasis placed on abstract concepts' that emerged in the latter years of schooling.[92] The situation was exacerbated by the fact that 'multiple [academic] failures . . . undermine individual children's ambition and causes a profound sense of failure and lack of motivation – facts hardly conducive to learning'.[93]

Such issues were particularly pertinent in the growing American slums. Conant's concerns about the drop-out rates in slum-area schools, 'where as many as half of the children drop out of school in grades 9, 10, and 11', might have reflected admirable aspirations, but also thrust a spotlight on the behavioural problems deemed to contribute to such rates.[94] Although Conant strongly advocated increased funding for such districts in order to improve high school completion rates, it became clear to many educators that hyperactivity was becoming an explanation for the academic under-achievement of slum-area children at the expense of social and economic explanations. To some, not enough effort was being taken to invest in 'the total environment of our children from inadequate homes and backgrounds'.[95]

Under pressure to attain higher school-completion rates, schools eagerly accepted labels such as hyperactivity as an explanation for why many of their students failed to succeed.[96] Some observers, such as psychologist Howard Adelman, accused schools of labelling failing students as disordered in order to salvage the school's reputation, arguing that 'whenever a youngster's learning problems can be attributed to deficits in the instructional process, that child should not be categorized as learning disabled'.[97] Others argued that in some cases, the 'possibility always exists that the managerial and programming skills of the adult may be as incompetent as the compliance skills of the child' and that there might be a need for a diagnosis of 'adults with programming disabilities, rather than one for children with learning disabilities'.[98] Although there might have been some truth in these assessments, it is also clear that the schools in the late 1950s and 1960s were in a difficult position. They were dealing with many more students, who were also expected to reach high levels of achievement, despite the fact that in previous decades they would have abandoned academic pursuits for unskilled labour. As students struggled to succeed in such conditions, the behaviours associated with their presumed underachievement were increasingly identified and diagnosed as hyperactivity.

The School Counsellor

Despite the concerns of Adelmen and others, American school-children during the 1960s were ever more diagnosed with hyper-activity. The disorder was increasingly seen as a key explanation for why children failed to achieve academic success. One important cog in the diagnostic machine was represented by a relatively new profession in American education, the school counsellor, funding for which was made possible by the NDEA. Counsellors played the role of mediator between the educational sphere, where hyperactive behaviour was increasingly recognized, and the medical sphere, where such behaviour was diagnosed as a disorder and treated. Education critics of the late 1950s were adamant that counsellors had an essential role in improving American education. Conant, for example, stressed the establishment of a comprehensive counselling infrastructure (at a student to counsellor ratio of 250:1) and believed counselling to be an essential part of any 'satisfactory' elementary or secondary school.[99] He especially called on school counsellors to

> be on the lookout for the bright boy or girl whose high ability has been demonstrated by the results of aptitude tests . . . but whose achievement, as measured by grades in courses, has been low.[100]

This description of the under-achieving student of average or above-average intelligence would become the stereotype of the hyper-active child.[101]

Historian Alexander Rippa has confirmed that many schools did follow Conant's recommendation, hiring large numbers of counsellors who specialized in identifying problems.[102] His view is reflected in education periodicals where it is also apparent that these counsellors were instrumental in identifying hyperactive, inattentive and impulsive children and viewing them as a discrete category of problem children, separate from the 'mentally retarded' and '"pure" emotionally disturbed'.[103] Teachers were also an important part of identifying such behaviours, for example by learning 'the difference between serious symptoms in child behaviour and simply annoying behaviour' – described elsewhere as 'one of the great psychiatric dilemmas of our time' – but were expected to cede responsibility for rehabilitating hyperactive, inattentive children to counselling staff.[104] While some teachers resented this intrusion into their domain, it was also believed that others sought 'diagnostic solace as a means of rationalizing her own programming inadequacies'. In other words, teachers unable to control the behaviour of hyperactive, impulsive children in their classroom were now able to rely on counsellors to determine 'some medical or psychological malady' and absolve themselves of blame for their student's difficulties.[105] According to Eric Denhoff, once counsellors and educators discovered that drugs such as Ritalin could help calm such children down, they 'began to encourage parents to seek such help from the child's physician'.[106] Despite Denhoff's advocacy of stimulant medication for hyperactive children, he feared that 'these drugs were being used indiscriminately – prescription would depend mostly upon a description of behaviour by a teacher or parent'.[107]

Whatever the teachers' motivations, the emergence of the counsellor as an additional resource in American schools undoubtedly facilitated the process by which problem students were labelled as hyperactive and referred for treatment. Although counsellors often recommended educational interventions, the low success rates of such measures compelled them to refer hyperactive students to physicians for medical treatment.[108] Indeed, counsellor John Peterson admitted that his colleagues sought 'a panacea for our non-performing students, a magic that will stir the laggard and salve the distressed'.[109] For many hyperactive children, the panacea provided by physicians was stimulant medications, such as Ritalin. In an era where scientific advancement was thought to take priority over everything, it was somehow appropriate that the solution for the problem of the hyperactive child, the symbol of American academic underachievement, was to be found in the highly scientific, highly technical setting of a pharmaceutical laboratory.

Although the US essentially ended the space race in 1969 by placing men on the moon, this triumph of American education ironically paralleled a tightening of federal education expenditure, as monies were instead allocated to fight the Vietnam War. The NDEA had won its primary objective of surpassing Soviet technological prowess, but returns were diminishing for many American students, especially those struggling to cope with raised expectations for academic and behavioural performance. Concern about hyperactivity remained, however, and even increased during the 1970s, as pharmaceutical companies, physicians and parent advocacy groups took the lead in condemning such behaviour and marketing pharmaceutical solutions.[110] As the Great Society education programmes faded from memory, hyperactivity and learning disabilities remained one of the few areas where government resources were still being directed.[111]

Much has changed in the US since the late 1950s, but many of the worries that spurred interest in hyperactivity then have re-emerged in the last decade. The US is once again involved in an intractable, divisive and ideological conflict, not with global communism, but with the equally problematic concept of 'terror'. Concurrently, American economic supremacy is under threat from China, India, Brazil and Russia. Fittingly, when the NDEA reached its fiftieth anniversary in 2008, fears about the United States' slipping position in the world spurred calls for a new such Act. The Association of American Universities warned that 'as the scientific and technological advantage that the U.S. has held over other nations is slipping away . . . [to] rapidly developing economies, particularly in Asia', a new Act was required 'to enhance the pipeline of U.S. students trained in fields vital to our national and economic security'.[112] The fields mentioned mimicked those identified in 1958, namely, 'science, mathematics, engineering and languages'. As during the Cold War, the geopolitical situation facing the US threatens to dictate education and, perhaps, mental health policy.

Many factors contributed to the emergence of hyperactivity as a ubiquitous phenomenon during the late 1950s. Hyperkinetic Impulse Disorder, which was transformed into Hyperkinetic Reaction of Childhood in DSM-II (1968) and then Attention Deficit Disorder in DSM-III (1980) provided a label that was extraordinarily easy to apply to countless children. Leaving Sputnik and education to one side, numerous other aspects of the filiarchal American society of the late 1950s and 1960s also likely contributed to the perception that numerous children had behavioural problems. These include changes to how children were disciplined (decreasing use of corporal punishment), how they spent their leisure time (watching television and listening to rock and roll instead of playing outside) and how children and youth increasingly challenged traditional American values (particularly those who became Beatniks and Hippies).

But underlying all such concerns was the fact that society's expectations of American children rose during this period, largely due to the pressures of the Cold War, but also because of how children were perceived more generally. Childhood, as seen through the philosophy of the American Association of Universities, along with their Cold War predecessors, is nothing more than a period of investment which is returned in the form of American national and economic security. As an American college professor put it in 1959, the Soviet education system was better because it served 'the purpose of the Soviet political and social system better than our system of education'.[113] Statements such as these provide evidence for the contention of sociologist Allan Horwitz that the desire to control children with disorders such as hyperactivity far outweighs the possibility that they have a specific pathology.[114] Similar thinking in the context of New Labour Britain has led historian Harry Hendrick to observe that

> children . . . are too valuable in terms of human capital to be given any say in shaping their own lives. Rather, they are to be possessed in order to maximise their potential as investments in our future.[115]

Although thinking of children as human capital might be excused as being sensibly utilitarian, this rationale, as Hendrick implies, obscures the fact that it is those in power, and not the disadvantaged members of the whole, who benefit from such accruement. In the case of hyperactivity this has also been the case, as the perceived needs of the state subsumed those of the child in the process of identifying certain behaviours as being pathological, and then attempting to medicate them out of existence.

THREE

Debating Hyperactivity

It is difficult to characterize psychiatry during the 1960s, the decade in which Laufer and Denhoff's hyperkinetic impulse disorder was transformed from a relatively unknown disorder to a condition worthy of entry into the canon of American psychiatry, DSM-II (1968), as 'hyperkinetic reaction of childhood (or adolescence).[1] If you had felt the need to visit a psychiatrist during the 1960s, the physician you saw could have come from one of any number of disparate ideological and clinical backgrounds. While the stereotypical image of the psychiatrist during the period was that of a psychoanalyst, rooted in Freudian philosophy, clutching a notebook and in the possession of a comfortable sofa, the development of new antipsychotic, antidepressant and other psychoactive drugs meant that a biological psychiatrist would have perceived your mental ills as a neurological problem and prescribed a pill instead of psychotherapy. In contrast, if you had happened to visit a psychiatrist at one of the many community mental health centres being built, it is likely that you would have been treated by a social psychiatrist, who would have looked to social problems, such as poverty, overcrowding and exposure to violence, as potential explanations for your troubles. Or, you might have also come across a much more sceptical psychiatrist, well versed in the antipsychiatry literature of Michel Foucault, R. D. Laing, Thomas Szasz and Erving Goffman, who would have judged any attempt to medicalize, let alone treat, variances in behaviour as an example of pernicious social control. Psychiatry in the 1960s could mean many things.

Given this context, it is not surprising that the psychiatric community had difficulty coming to a consensus about hyperactivity. Psychiatrists disagreed about what caused the disorder, whether it was permanent or developmental and how best to treat it. These tensions were exacerbated during the post-war period by the perception that mental illness was rife in American society and that it was the responsibility of psychiatrists to solve the problem. Spurred on by politicians, most notably President John F. Kennedy (1917–1963), psychiatrists were called upon to address the United States' mental health woes, but psychoanalysts, social psychiatrists and biological psychiatrists had difficulty agreeing about how to do so. At stake for these competing approaches was not only the nation's mental health and the prestige of psychiatry, but also the dominance of the profession itself.

It is difficult to see how the competing explanations and solutions for mental illness could have been more different. While psychoanalysts saw insanity as a manifestation of unresolved childhood conflicts that were best addressed through psychotherapy, biological psychiatrists believed mental illness was caused by genetic or organic neurological dysfunction and was best treated by drugs. Often forgotten today, social psychiatrists looked to the social origins of mental illness and argued that such problems could be prevented by alleviating inequality in society.

The manner in which DSM-II dealt with hyperactivity underlined such divisions.[2] Although its authorship was dominated by psychoanalysts, it was difficult for hyperactivity to be viewed in solely psychodynamic terms. This was because of the history of associating hyperactive behaviour with brain damage, caused by infections and brain injury, and reflected in terms such as post-encephalitic disorder, organic drivenness and minimal brain damage. Because of this, hyperactivity was not only mentioned in terms of hyperkinetic reaction of childhood, in the broader category of 'behavior disorders of childhood and adolescence', but also in the category of non-psychotic organic brain syndromes. As mentioned in chapter One, hyperactivity was only one of a number of behavioural symptoms linked to brain damage and the authors of DSM-II noted that children so affected could also be 'withdrawn', 'listless' and 'unresponsive' as well as psychotic.[3] Despite the inclusion of organic conditions, the psychoanalytical orientation of the manual was made clear by the assertion that if these children's symptoms were dominated by negative interactions with their parents, then they should be given a 'behavior disorder' diagnosis rather than one based on organic brain syndrome. In other words, 'interactional factors', specifically the child's relationship with his/her parents, were more important in terms of diagnosis than evidence of brain damage.[4]

The term hyperkinetic reaction of childhood similarly reflected psychoanalytical thinking, but also suggested a psychosocial aspect due to the use of the term 'reaction'. Reactions were seen as responses to particular experiences or events, which could be social in nature, in addition to being caused by interactional problems within the family. The other 'reactions' listed, including those associated with withdrawing, running away, anxiety, aggression and delinquency, likewise invoked a social dimension.[5] The developmental nature of hyperkinetic reaction of childhood was also stressed, as it was believed to affect young children most and often diminished during adolescence. According to DSM-II, hyperactivity was a symptom common to a number of disorders and could be triggered by biological, social or psychodynamic causes.

This apparently pluralistic approach to hyperactivity belied the interdisciplinary squabbles that plagued psychiatry before and after DSM-II's publication. Almost as soon as the manual was published, biological psychiatrists, including Richard L. Jenkins, the chair of the committee who wrote DSM-III, began expressing concerns about its psychodynamic leanings.[6] At stake in these debates was not only the future of American psychiatry, but also how disorders like hyperactivity would be understood and treated, as well as how those diagnosed with mental disorders saw themselves and their afflictions. Underlying such tensions was psychiatry's long-held desire to be seen as an authoritative medical science. As historian Charles E. Rosenberg has explained, American psychiatry was often seen by those both within and outside the discipline as existing on the low rung of the medical ladder, at best, and a quasi-medical science at worst.[7] As the reviewer of a book on child psychiatry described:

'Bold is the physician who leaves the safe havens of general medicine for the less well charted waters of psychiatry, a prey to clutching at superstitions and half truths.'[8]

Psychiatry's fraught position was due in large part to the socially contingent nature of what was considered mental illness; as society changed, so too did notions of what was sane and insane. Making matters worse was the fact that, as Roy Porter and Mark S. Micale have described, psychiatric theories could differ drastically from one another. While some psychiatrists believed that mental illness was purely neurological and advocated treatments ranging from lobotomies and drugs to electro and insulin shock therapy, others stressed the dynamic nature of mental health and preferred talking therapies such as psychoanalysis.[9] Such discrepancies did not endear psychiatrists to the broader American medical community, which sought to professionalize and standardize medical education. Whereas Freudian and Jungian theories of medical illness could be seen as more philosophy than science, treatments such as lobotomy could be seen as an example of heroic medicine gone a step too far.[10] Psychiatrists also had to contest the notion, which had been accurate to a point, that they were little more than asylum superintendents, responsible for warehousing society's abnormal and unwanted. Concerns about how patients were treated in such facilities, as well as doubts about the validity of mental illness itself, gave rise to the anti-psychiatry movement during the late 1950s and 1960s, as writers, philosophers, sociologists, historians and psychiatrists themselves questioned the mission and purpose of psychiatry.[11] Perhaps most importantly, mental illness was and is extraordinarily difficult to treat, let alone cure or prevent. While developments in antibiotics, cardiac surgery and chemotherapy during the 1940s gave hope to the patients of internists, cardiologists and oncologists, thus increasing the prestige of such disciplines, their mentally ill counterparts were faced with the prospect of institutionalization, psychosurgery, shock therapy or expensive and time-consuming psychoanalysis. In comparison to other specialties, psychiatry's development appeared to be sporadic, meandering and oftentimes regressive. Given its unpromising outlook, it is not surprising that some medical students who opted to specialize in psychiatry were thought to be somewhat unbalanced themselves.[12]

Despite this ongoing sense of crisis, however, American psychiatrists also had many reasons to be optimistic at the end of the Second World War. Chief among these was that, anti-psychiatry notwithstanding, many influential Americans believed that the United States was suffering from escalating levels of mental illness and looked to psychiatry for solutions. Concerns about mental health were prompted by the high numbers of Americans who were rejected for military service on psychiatric grounds during the war, but was also fuelled by the ambitions of the profession itself. Leaders within psychiatry, such as Robert Felix (1904–1985), were keen to put mental health at the centre of public health policy.[13] This not only involved a shift away from caring for the mentally ill in asylums and towards community care and prevention, but also a transition away from the neuropsychiatric paradigm, which prevailed in such institutions, and towards a more psychodynamic approach. The rise of psychoanalysis was also associated with both the large number of influential American psychiatrists who travelled to Europe to study the subject and the flight of psychoanalysts from Nazi Germany to North America.[14]

Felix and others, including William Menninger (1899–1966), who headed the neuropsychiatry section of the Surgeon General's office during the Second World War, were able to convince the American government that the 'eradication and prevention' of mental illness, 'one of mankind's greatest afflictions', was not only vital, it was also possible.[15] In 1946 such ambitions were instilled in the National Mental Health Act, which led to the creation of the National Institutes of Mental Health (NIMH) with Felix at its head.[16] Seeking to establish a new theoretical and political framework to combat mental illness, the 1946 Act was followed up by the Mental Health Study Act (1955), modelled on the report tabled by Abraham Flexner in 1910 in an effort to revolutionize medical education.[17] The 1955 Act led to the creation of the Joint Commission on Mental Illness and Health (JCMIH), which was tasked to conduct 'an objective, thorough, nationwide analysis and re-evaluation of the human and economic problems of mental health'. The JCMIH's final report, *Action for Mental Health* (1961), was 'a sweeping document that spelled out a vision of the future', a call to action on many fronts to combat mental illness, with psychiatrists leading the charge.[18]

Children were of particular concern to the JCMIH and soon the Joint Commission on the Mental Health of Children (JCMHC) was created to address the 'groundswell of pressure for a study on the mental health needs of children'.[19] The JCMHC's findings also stressed how children's mental health was crucial in the larger struggle against mental illness. As one commentator described, it is 'unlikely that history has seen so bold and encompassing a statement on the needs and rights of children'.[20] Burgeoning interest in children's mental health was also evidenced by the founding of the *Journal of the American Academy of Child Psychiatry* (JAACP) in 1962.

Psychiatry also received a boost from President Kennedy, who incorporated a mental health agenda into his Great Frontier policies. In his Message to Congress on Mental Health and Mental Retardation (1963), Kennedy argued that

> infectious epidemics are now largely under control. Most of the major diseases of the body are beginning to give ground in man's increasing struggle to find their cause and cure. But the public understanding, treatment and prevention of mental disabilities have not made comparable progress since the earliest days of modern history.[21]

Congress was moved enough by Kennedy's speech to pass the Community Mental Health Center's Construction Act in 1963.[22] Leaders within the psychiatric community, especially following the president's assassination, were also compelled to address Kennedy's 'dramatic and heart-warming' interest in mental illness. According to C. H. Hardin Branch, president of the American Psychiatric Association (APA) in 1962–3, the psychiatric profession needed 'men – and women – to match the mountains of opportunity now arising out of the plains of apathy and disinterest'.[23] The Council of the APA agreed, stating that Kennedy had been the

first president of the United States to champion the cause
of the mentally ill ... It must be our faith that the realization
of the President's dream of a wholly new approach to mental illness would abate the very violence which struck him
down. It must be our tribute to him that we quicken our
resolve to make that dream come true.[24]

American psychiatry did face 'mountains of opportunity' but
just how the discipline should deal with the challenge of solving
the nation's mental health problems was unclear. The history of
hyperactivity during the 1960s and 1970s demonstrates how, far
from adopting the pluralistic approach suggested by Kennedy,
psychoanalysts, social psychiatrists and biological psychiatrists
attempted to eclipse one another in order to dominate the
profession. Biological psychiatrists emerged victorious out of this
struggle and their genetic and neurological explanations of and
psychopharmaceutical treatments for hyperactivity, and other
mental disorders, prevailed from the 1970s onwards. The reasons
why this was the case has partly to do with the fact that the biological approach to hyperactivity was less expensive, time-consuming
and complicated than that of its rivals, but also because it was best
suited to adapt to the ideological, technological and political
changes within psychiatry itself.

Psychoanalysis: 'Productive and Cohesive'

Psychoanalysis emerged out of the Second World War as the dominant discipline within American psychiatry, taking over the mantle
previously held by asylum-based biological psychiatrists.[25] The
growth of psychoanalysis in the United States was due to a number
of factors, including a shift from the asylum to the private clinic as
the locus of mental health treatment and the influx of Jewish psychoanalysts from Europe during the 1930s and 1940s. The discipline
influenced both clinical practice and research, as well as how the
public perceived psychiatry and psychiatrists.[26] The image of the
patient on a couch, relating his or her childhood experiences, while
a well-dressed psychoanalyst thoughtfully took notes, became one

of psychiatry's enduring symbols, reflecting an intellectual and sophisticated, but also somewhat detached and unemotional, approach to treatment.

Psychoanalysis was also an influential political force within psychiatry. Many psychoanalysts took up the presidency of the APA, headed university departments and held other prestigious posts during the post-war period, leading the profession through a turbulent, yet also promising period, and psychoanalytical thought prevailed especially in child psychiatry.[27] The JAACP, for instance, was edited by psychoanalyst Eveoleen N. Rexford and, accordingly, most of the articles the journal published during the 1960s were psychoanalytically oriented. In a special series on childhood behavioural problems in 1963, for example, all of the articles were based in psychoanalytic theory.[28] To many, psychoanalysis was the 'most productive and cohesive theory available'.[29]

Not all psychiatrists, however, were happy with this state of affairs and, conscious of their critics, psychoanalysts defended their hegemony over American psychiatry vigorously, increasingly so as rival theories became popular. A letter written by Iowa child psychiatrist Mark A. Stewart to the editor of the American Journal of Psychiatry (AJP) in 1960, for instance, highlighted their dominance, but also implied that not all psychiatrists were happy with the situation. Stewart stated that jobs advertised in the APA's 'Mail Pouch' nearly always stressed the importance of a psychoanalytic orientation and complained that 'this phenomenon, which unhappily is symptomatic of the general situation of psychiatry today, can make our profession seem ridiculous to other physicians and scientists in general'.[30] Despite Stewart's criticism, for many psychiatrists working during the emergence of hyperactivity, mental health had little to do with neurology; there was no 'magical belief in some kind of correspondence between psychical processes and central nervous processes'.[31]

This lack of faith or even interest in neurological explanations for mental illness was reflected in psychoanalytical explanations for hyperactivity. According to psychoanalysts, hyperactivity was rooted in familial dynamics and involved disruption of the superego which, in turn, resulted in poor impulse control.[32] Although this explanation appeared simple superficially, the key for psychoanalysis was to determine what initially caused such disruption in order to provide effective psychotherapy. Two aspects of this approach to hyperactivity made psychoanalysts particularly vulnerable to criticism. First, psychoanalysts stressed the uniqueness of each hyperactive patient and his or her specific course of therapy. No magic bullets were promised. As such, psychoanalysis required a great deal of faith in its efficacy and a substantial degree of patience on the part of both clinician and patient. Second, psychoanalysts described hyperactivity as a distinctly mental, as opposed to neurological, phenomenon. Drugs were only helpful in that they might lead to better psychotherapy in some patients.[33]

With such an emphasis on the individual patient, most of the psychoanalytic articles published during the 1960s about hyperactivity were written in the form of case studies featuring the clinical observations of a single patient. The patient would be introduced along with a detailed description of his or her behaviours, personality, history and family situation. The authors would then describe how they were able to unravel the reasons for the patient's hyperactivity and recount the course of treatment. In a 1960 issue of the journal *Archives of General Psychiatry*, for example, the story of 'Jean' was told. Jean was a twelve-year-old girl whose impulsive behaviour, her psychiatrist determined, was the result of penis envy stemming from the relationship she had with her father. Jean's impulsivity ceased only when she was able to come to terms with this explanation.[34] The root causes of hyperactivity in other children could also originate in the child's weaning, toilet training, adjustment to a new sibling or other types of trauma.[35] In other cases, inappropriate, unhealthy or inadequate relationships with parents were believed to be the problem.[36]

In many ways, case studies were an attractive means by which to depict hyperactivity and course of psychoanalytic treatment. The reader was provided with a narrative which usually resulted in a happy ending; the child who was so disruptive at the beginning was usually thriving at both school and home by the end. Although sceptics could question the reliability of such descriptions, case studies had an emotional impact upon readers which the impersonal accounts of double-blind clinical trials lacked. The patients were real children, not anonymous numbers, and the clinicians were presented as detectives of the mind, seeking out the source of such trouble with a combination of insight, deduction and compassion.

But despite the success stories depicted in such case studies, the psychoanalytic approach to hyperactivity was also heavily criticized. For parents of hyperactive children, psychoanalytic explanations of their children's behaviour were often confusing and contradictory, and seemed to imply, if not explicitly state, that they were to blame. Mothers were singled out in particular, fitting into larger trends in child guidance.[37] As Barbara Ehrenreich and Deirdre English have described, 'by the mid-twentieth century the experts were grimly acknowledging that despite constant vigilance the American mother was failing at her job'. Mothers were accused of being overindulgent in one moment and then inattentive the next.[38]

Other psychiatric theories not only absolved mothers of blame, but also provided exciting new therapies. Drugs such as the antipsychotic Thorazine and the antidepressant Miltown were advertised as being able to help patients ranging from the institutionalized schizophrenic to the depressed housewife. As pharmaceutical companies began experiencing success selling such drugs during the 1950s and 1960s, psychoanalysis was increasingly seen as anachronistic and unscientific, particularly by those who desired to see psychiatry gain the respect of other medical disciplines.[39] Many believed that psychoanalysis should be the remit of social workers and psychologists, not medically trained psychiatrists. As child psychiatrist John S. Werry described, encouraging his colleagues to employ 'pediatric psychopharmacology', 'child psychiatry . . . is not simply a humanitarian exercise, but an applied medical science'.[40]

Some writers, particularly Jonathan Metzl, have argued that Freudian ideas about gender and sex remained inherent in how psychoactive drugs were designed, marketed and prescribed, suggesting that the line between psychoanalytic and biological approaches to psychiatry was somewhat blurred. Medications geared towards reinforcing gender roles, contends Metzl, replaced male psychoanalysts who were intent on doing the same.[41] To a degree, this is true. Gender norms, either imbued with or free from Freudian subtext, certainly can be read into psychiatric drug advertisements of the 1960s and 1970s, but it could also be argued that advertisements for hyperactivity drugs, targeted chiefly at boys, undermined many gendered ideas about the rambunctious, active and assertive manner in which boys were expected to act. Boys who were made of frogs and snails and puppy dog tails, in other words, were liable to cause trouble and end up on Ritalin. Metzl's gender argument, however valid in the cases of some medications and disorders, does not eclipse the fact that most biological psychiatrists saw themselves as being diametrically opposed to psychoanalysis. Scientifically, clinically and philosophically, biological psychiatrists like John Werry believed they were operating in a completely different psychiatric paradigm.

Psychoanalysts, it must be said, often felt the same about their biologically oriented colleagues. Despite the excitement and sales generated by the new medications, however, many psychoanalysts insisted that neurology and psychiatry should not mix. As Albert J. Solnit (1919–2002), one of the first American child psychiatrists, asserted, 'there is considerable doubt that the use of research models derived from the physical sciences can be of more than limited usefulness in child psychiatry research'.[42] Solnit's assertion generated a heated response from Leon Eisenberg (1922–2009), who had conducted the first large-scale Ritalin trials with C. Keith Conners. Eisenberg stated that psychoanalysis had a 'constricting influence' on psychiatry and that the case studies published in journals such as JAACP should be replaced with 'epidemiological, pharmacological, and psychological studies'.[43]

The practicality of providing psychotherapy to the vast numbers of hyperactive children, variably estimated at between 3 and 20 per cent of the childhood population, was also questioned.[44] Psychoanalytic theory required that each case be treated individually, or in the words of one psychoanalyst, 'individual psychotherapy is the only treatment that roots out the trouble. You can't apply this on a mass basis.'[45] Critics such as Eisenberg countered that there were 'more people struggling in the stream of life than we can rescue with our present tactics' of using psychoanalysis.[46] Others claimed simply that there were nowhere near enough psychotherapists to treat the 'extraordinary numbers of disturbed children in the country', meaning that 'the vast majority of children needing clinical care do not receive it'.[47] Although group therapy was becoming a popular strategy, the practicalities of offering such measures to hyperactive children precluded it from becoming an alternative, despite some attempts.[48]

The effectiveness of psychotherapy in treating hyperactivity altogether was also doubted by some. Writing in the *Journal of the American Medical Association* (JAMA), Harold B. Levy charged that 'unfortunate children with minimal brain dysfunction are still being condemned to months of fruitless and frustrating psychotherapy in various guidance clinics, while guilt and resentment builds upon their bewildered parents'.[49] He proceeded to claim that 'misdirected psychotherapy can be every bit as dangerous as misdirected surgery'.[50] While this specific charge might have been overly polemical, psychoanalysts themselves admitted that psychotherapy could be a time-consuming, expensive and emotionally demanding intervention.[51] It was also difficult for psychoanalysts to prove the effectiveness of psychotherapy in the manner increasingly expected by medical researchers, namely, double-blind randomly controlled trials. Biological psychiatrists, in contrast, used the results from their trials of stimulant drugs extremely effectively to convince their colleagues, educators and parents that products such as Ritalin could improve the behaviour of hyperactive children.

Even psychoanalysts who were confident about the efficacy of psychotherapy generally could nonetheless find that their hyperactive patients posed a therapeutic challenge. Psychotherapy required that a patient concentrate, be reflective and follow dutifully the psychotherapist's suggestions. Understandably, this was an arduous requirement for hyperactive children to meet. One psychoanalyst described how her patient's 'hyperactivity increased and all in a matter of a few minutes, she sat on my desk, wrote on the blackboard, and picked her nose excessively'.[52] Unsurprisingly, she was unable to help the patient and proceeded to suggest that this was an indication that her patient's hyperactivity was due to neurological damage. It is somewhat strange that psychoanalysts did not suggest play therapy more often, employed as early as 1926 by Anna

Freud (1895–1982), as a possible intervention for hyperactive children.[53] Freud saw play therapy as a means to strengthen ego functioning by encouraging children to verbalize what they were feeling at play. Within the bounds of psychoanalytic theory, such therapy would have presumably provided some insights into what drove the impulsivity of the hyperactive child, but was rarely attempted.[54]

The challenges of providing psychotherapy to hyperactive children led many psychiatrists to go as far as to accuse psychoanalysts of turning away hyperactive children from their practices.[55] Whether or not this was the case, it was clear that very few families could afford the time, money or patience required for psychoanalysis. The combination of practical difficulties, emerging alternatives and growing dissatisfaction with the apparently unscientific nature of psychoanalysis meant that psychotherapy never became a popular treatment for hyperactivity. When a non-pharmaceutical option was offered during the 1970s, it tended to be behaviour therapy rather than psychoanalysis. Psychoanalytic explanations for hyperactivity might have helped to explain some aspects of the disorder, but as psychiatrists increasingly looked to neurological approaches to mental illness, it failed to remain a viable treatment alternative.

Social Psychiatry: 'A Preventive Psychiatry'

If President Kennedy's 1963 Message to Congress is any indication, social psychiatry seemed poised to challenge psychoanalysis for dominance in psychiatry. Kennedy's emphasis on eliminating the environmental causes of mental illness, especially poverty, mirrored the preventive strategies of social psychiatry:

> we must seek out the causes of mental illness and of mental retardation and eradicate them. Here, more than in any other area, 'an ounce of prevention is worth more than a pound of cure.' For prevention is far more desirable for all concerned. It is far more economical and it is far more likely to be successful. Prevention will require both selected specific programs directed especially at known causes, and the general strengthening of our fundamental community,

social welfare, and educational programs which can do much to eliminate or correct the harsh environmental conditions which often are associated with mental retardation and mental illness.[56]

Kennedy also stressed less reliance on institutionalizing patients, which he called 'social quarantine', and instead a shift towards more numerous, smaller and local community mental health centres, another tenet of social psychiatry. Following Kennedy's assassination by Lee Harvey Oswald in late 1963, Congress passed the Community Mental Health Centers Construction Act (nicknamed the 'Oswald Bill' due to the belief that the Act might have prevented Oswald's actions; indeed a *Life* article suggested that Oswald was hyperactive), which helped to realize some of the president's ambitions.[57] While biological psychiatrists and psychoanalysts facilitated this move, by providing drugs and counselling, the new community focus rested on the foundations of social psychiatry.

Social psychiatrists were among the most outspoken critics of the individualized psychoanalytic approach to hyperactivity and offered their own, presumably more pragmatic solution. During the 1950s and 1960s, psychiatrists became increasingly concerned with preventing mental illness and, rather than looking at the brain or interfamilial dynamics, turned to society as the primary source of psychiatric problems. Building on the work of Robert L. Faris and H. Warren Dunham in Chicago during the 1930s, psychiatrists and sociologists, such as August B. Hollingshead, Fredrick C. Redlich, Leo Srole and Alexander Leighton worked together to explore the social determinants of mental health in communities ranging from rural Nova Scotia to midtown Manhattan.[58] For some social psychiatrists, mental illness could be prevented by alleviating its social causes, such as class inequalities, poverty, overcrowding, crime, prostitution and substance abuse. For others, social psychiatry was more concerned with providing psychiatric services in local areas to the people who needed them the most, the poor and downtrodden in society. It was the psychiatrist's duty, therefore, to get involved politically and fight to eliminate such pathogenic conditions. Psychiatrists were expected to advocate for public housing projects, improved schools and employment programmes in order to prevent mental illness among society's disadvantaged.[59] In many ways, the social psychiatrist's role was as political as it was medical.

Despite its seemingly radical aims, the prophylactic strategies espoused by social psychiatrists reflected the beliefs of many psychiatrists during the 1960s, as well as the official policy of the APA, especially with respect to children.[60] One of the reasons for this was that social psychiatric theory, while it reflected many of the socially progressive ideals of the 1960s, was also utilitarian. Kennedy himself had stated that his arguments in favour of preventive psychiatry were based on both compassion and utility.[61] Such thinking was also reflected in the views of many of the presidents of the APA during the 1960s, who urged their colleagues to study the pathological effects of social problems.[62] Much as the founding of JAACP was in response to growing concern about the mental health of children, the *International Journal of Social Psychiatry* (IJSP) and *Social Psychiatry* were founded in 1956 and 1966 respectively to reflect interest in preventive mental health. The editorial statement which graced the inaugural edition of *Social Psychiatry* not only stressed how such journals would 'disseminate this growing body of pertinent knowledge', but also emphasized that the 'world-wide movement toward a social orientation affects psychiatric practice, education and research'. The statement proceeded to describe the editors' interest in papers that reported 'on the social, cultural and familial determinants of psychic disorders and their implications for social and psychological treatment'.[63]

As Sir David Henderson (1884–1965), British psychiatrist and professor of psychiatry at the University of Edinburgh, indicated in his letter supporting the founding of IJSP, social psychiatry also had its roots in previous generations of psychiatrists, including the work of Adolph Meyer (1866–1950) during the first decades of the twentieth century in New York. Henderson went on to stress that

> social psychiatry is first and foremost a preventative psychiatry. It strives to combat all those causes of social and environmental nature which are manageable and it concerns itself with public welfare in the widest sense.[64]

A letter writer in a subsequent issue put matters more bluntly, stating that 'social life is a prolific breeder of mental disease', and that 'we would do, both for the patient and for society as a whole, immediately better if we could go to the roots of these troubles'. Among the pernicious social factors listed were long working hours, poverty, war, racial discrimination and segregation.[65]

Taken in the context of the 1960s, in the midst of the 'New Frontier' and 'Great Society' policy initiatives of Presidents Kennedy and Johnson, the civil rights movement and protests against the Vietnam War, it was understandable that many psychiatrists were interested in the preventive concepts of social psychiatry. Support for a social approach to mental illness emanated from other sources as well. Books such as Michael Harrington's (1928–1989) The Other America (1962), which argued that up to a quarter of Americans lived in poverty, sold over a million copies and helped to inspire President Johnson's 'War on Poverty', added an urgency to the claims of social psychiatrists.[66] The work of Montreal-based endocrinologist Hans Selye (1907–1982), whose general adaptation syndrome provided a physiological rationale for linking social stressors and illness, also helped substantiate the link between social deprivation and mental disorder.[67] Children were understandably a key focus for social psychiatrists and it did not take long for research to indicate that social factors played a role in disorders such as hyperactivity. Studies began to demonstrate that children brought up in poverty and exposed to vices such as petty crime, prostitution and violence were much more likely to be hyperactive, impulsive and inattentive in school and succumb to mental illness later on in life.[68] Such conclusions reflected the contention in a 'Medical News' column in JAMA that 30 per cent of children in deprived areas required psychiatric help.[69] Influential child psychiatrists Stella Chess (1914–2007), Alexander Thomas (1914–2003), Michael Rutter (b. 1933) and Herbert G. Birch (1918–1973) similarly claimed that environmental factors could cause childhood behavioural disorders such as hyperactivity.[70] Other researchers found that hyperactivity was most commonly diagnosed in poor children, often representing visible minorities.[71]

Even some biologically oriented psychiatrists, such Leon Eisenberg, were sympathetic to social psychiatric ideas. Eisenberg's research on stimulants and hyperactivity at Johns Hopkins University during the 1960s proved to be an influential catalyst for a tremendous amount of subsequent neuropsychiatric research into hyperactivity. Despite his focus on pharmacotherapy, Eisenberg also believed that the 'severe and chronic deprivation experienced by the pre-delinquent child can only be dealt with by large scale forceful community efforts'.[72] He not only lamented that psychiatrists 'neglected prevention in our preoccupation with treatment', but also believed that 'much of the difficult behavior seen in association with brain damage syndrome [a synonym for hyperactivity] stems not from the anatomical deficits, but from the social consequences of personality development'.[73] Psychiatrists, according to Eisenberg, could and should be a powerful lobby that addressed a variety of social problems.[74]

Similarly, many psychoanalysts believed that the anxieties associated with poverty made children more susceptible to ego dysfunction and subsequent problems like hyperactivity.[75] Psychoanalyst Eleanor Pavenstedt, for instance, stressed the need for more research on the effects of poverty, substance abuse, prostitution, violence and crime on ego development.[76] Likewise, Charles A. Malone believed that 'disorganized' family situations characterized by brutality, alcoholism, illegitimacy, crime, delinquency and neglect led to 'acting out', a term often used by psychoanalysts to describe hyperactive behaviour. Malone believed that in the 'normless world', impulses like petty crime, prostitution, public urination and fighting were not only fantasized by children, but actually carried out.[77]

The JCMHC also emphasized that eliminating the socio-economic hardships faced by children was a key factor in preventing mental illness. Reginald S. Lourie, who headed the Commission, was willing to 'recommend a radical reconstruction of the present system in order to solve the mental health problems of children'.[78] The APA agreed, saying that the recommendations of the JCMHC would 'strengthen the nation's resolve and capacity to deal with its awesome problems'.[79] Joseph D. Noshpitz, an associate editor for JAACP, echoed the APA's plea to American national interest by contending that the mental health priorities of children should be the government's primary commitment.[80] Even outside observers, such as Judge David L. Bazelon, who served on the JCMHC, concurred that the mental health needs of children were best served by providing healthy homes and improved schools.[81]

Ultimately, however, the bold social psychiatric agenda fell short of its lofty goals. Although the socio-economic solutions put forth by social psychiatrists garnered a great deal of support during the 1960s, and were reflected in legislation and in research activities, they nevertheless required more political fortitude than psychiatrists could muster, especially after federal funding shifted from the New Frontier and Great Society programmes to waging the war in Vietnam. Indicative of this trend was Henry W. Brosin's 'Presidential Address' to the APA in 1968/9. In his 'Response to the Presidential Address', the previous year, Brosin was optimistic about the prospects of reducing poverty and subsequently improving mental health.[82] A year later, his comments were less sanguine. He noted that American involvement in Vietnam was drawing resources away from mental health programmes and that difficult choices must be made regarding the direction of psychiatry's efforts.[83] Quoting John Gardner, the Secretary for Health, Education and Welfare, Brosin indicated that a 'crunch between expectations and resources' was occurring, especially with regards to 'early childhood education, work with handicapped children, special education for the disadvantaged'.[84]

Social psychiatry's approach to preventing hyperactivity, and other mental disorders, was ambitious, idealistic and revolutionary, requiring an enormous amount of political, social and economic change at all levels of government and society. Unfortunately, as Solnit noted, politicians, not psychiatrists, had the power to prevent the environmental causes of mental illness. Reflecting on how contemporary psychiatrists felt about social psychiatry, he (quoting poet Robert Lowell) admitted that

> One side of me is a conventional liberal, concerned with causes, agitated with peace and justice, and equality . . . My other side is deeply conservative, wanting to get at the root of things.[85]

Although social psychiatrists could argue that they were getting 'at the root of things', it was also true that while many psychiatrists believed that improving social conditions was a noble and potentially utilitarian psychiatric strategy, most were unwilling to commit as fully to the prophylactic prescription as social psychiatrists demanded. Those concerned about psychiatry's medical status also feared that social psychiatry's stress on socio-economic conditions, not to mention its endorsement of cooperation between psychiatry and other health professions, would damage psychiatry's always tenuous reputation.[86] Similarly, many psychiatrists disputed the notion that they should get involved in politics altogether.[87] Finally there were those who argued that social psychiatry's stress on alleviating poverty was simplistic, naïve and unlikely to work.[88]

The shortcomings of social psychiatry were also highlighted by disorders like hyperactivity. Social psychiatry's focus on prevention did little for children currently experiencing academic and social difficulties due to their behavioural problems. Socio-economic inequality might indeed cause much strife, and might even cause mental illness, but it did not entirely explain why disorders like hyperactivity occurred in both lower- and middle-class populations.[89] Despite Kennedy's endorsement, APA sympathy and the appeal of its preventive philosophy, social psychiatrists had difficulty addressing the escalating rates of disorders such as hyperactivity and, by the 1970s, psychiatrists and parents were looking to more immediate solutions.

Biological Psychiatry: 'A Twisted Molecule'

The field of psychiatry which seemed most able to provide the instantaneous response to hyperactivity demanded by psychiatrists and parents was biological psychiatry. Drawing on a long tradition of viewing mental illness as a predominantly neurological phenomenon, biological psychiatrists during the 1960s and 1970s were buoyed by recent advancements in pharmacology, particularly the development of psychoactive drugs. Soon most psychiatrists would believe that there was 'no twisted thought without a twisted molecule'.[90] With regards to hyperactivity, biological psychiatrists looked to the brain and its functioning for the causes of the disorder, and prescribed not only stimulant drugs, but also tranquillizers and antidepressants.[91] For many psychiatrists, biological psychiatry's emphasis on the neurological causes of mental illness gave the profession renewed respectability, something they believed was lacking during the years when psychoanalysis dominated.[92]

Biological psychiatry was also able to point to a tradition, dating back especially to the post-encephalitic disorder epidemic of the 1920s, of viewing childhood behaviour disorders as neurological phenomena. As such, many psychiatrists continue to refer to hyperactivity as minimal brain damage or dysfunction long after the emergence of terms such as hyperkinetic impulse disorder or hyperkinetic reaction of childhood. They could also claim, by highlighting the work of Charles Bradley during the late 1930s, that there was a history of treating disturbed children with stimulants. The first significant trial of Ritalin by Eisenberg and Conners in 1963, for example, pointed to the work of Bradley and some of his followers.[93]

Biological psychiatrists made key allies in pharmaceutical companies such as CIBA, the manufacturers of Ritalin, which were understandably interested in taking advantage of, if not exaggerating, the perceived hyperactivity epidemic. Not only did CIBA fund research and conferences on hyperactivity, they also produced films and pamphlets about the disorder and marketed it at Parent Teacher Association (PTA) meetings during the late 1960s and early 1970s.[94] Such marketing not only helps to explain the rise in hyperactivity rates, but also hints at why Ritalin became 'the treatment of choice [despite] . . . very little empirical basis for its supposed superiority' to other drugs such as dextroamphetamine.[95] Although the Convention on Psychotropic Substances in 1971 somewhat curtailed the practice of marketing directly to parents and teachers, physicians remained the target of drug companies, as pharmaceutical advertising in medical journals increased enormously during the 1960s and 1970s. As historian David Herzberg has observed, pharmaceutical companies also sponsored medical conferences, including one in 1964 which celebrated 'ten years of minor tranquilizers' and had its proceedings reprinted in the *Journal of Neuropsychiatry*.[96]

The use of stimulants reflected a larger trend in psychiatry towards pharmacotherapy, as historians such as Herzberg, Andrea Tone, Nicolas Rasmussen and others have discussed.[97] A quick look through the pages of JAMA during the 1960s and 1970s also indicates that the marketing of psychoactive drugs was not only widespread, but also aggressive, featuring creative, full-page advertisements that graphically depicted the horrors of mental illness and the benefits of drugs. One such advertisement featured a gaunt, exhausted PhD student whose thesis is described as being 'in progress'. The solution to the stress he feels, with which any PhD student would identify, was a prescription for Valium. The advertisement's message, that the strain of the student's intensive study could be alleviated by Valium, was directed both at physicians, who might recall similar stresses from their student days, and PhD and MD students who might have cause to look through JAMA for their research. Higher learning, according to Valium's manufacturers, could be a pathological activity.[98] By the early 1960s, in fact, some psychiatrists were complaining about the extent to which they were 'bombarded' with advertising by pharmaceutical companies.[99] Accordingly, a few journals, including the psychoanalytically oriented JAACP, refrained from running advertisements until much later.

Other factors were also crucial to the acceptance of biological interpretations of hyperactivity. By treating hyperactivity as a genetic, neurological condition, biological psychiatrists abandoned the tradition, implicit in both psychoanalytic and social psychiatric approaches, of blaming parents, usually mothers, for their children's mental health problems. As sociologist Ilina Singh has noted: 'weary of mother-blame . . . for mothers with problem boys, the news about drug treatment and the emphasis on the organic nature of children's behaviour problems appears to have been very welcome'.[100] The immediacy of Ritalin's effects was also compelling. Whereas Maurice Laufer was impressed with how quickly Ritalin worked, his colleague Eric Denhoff believed that Ritalin's efficacy was such that he considered 'it as "sort of criminal" to withhold treatment from those who can use it'.[101]

Although some biological psychiatrists were puzzled by the fact that stimulants seemed paradoxically to calm hyperactive children, the belief in their effectiveness was such that, in some cases, stimulants were used as a diagnostic tool: if they calmed down an overactive, impulsive child, then the child likely had hyperactivity.[102] More importantly for parents, however, was that stimulants were a quicker, easier and less expensive treatment modality than arranging for psychotherapy or analysing and attempting to change the social factors that might be contributing to such behaviour. Such drugs appeared to be veritable magic bullets.

As the next chapter contends, it would be a mistake to believe that Ritalin was the wonder drug the advertisements portrayed. Its effects were nearly instantaneous, but the drug did not cure or prevent hyperactivity; it only controlled the symptoms temporarily. Stimulants worked for only 80 per cent of patients and their effectiveness faded with time, requiring higher dosages to be prescribed.[103] With millions of diagnosed children, 20 per cent amounted to a substantial population of untreated patients. Biological psychiatrists also downplayed the side effects of Ritalin, including growth inhibition, irritability, insomnia, anorexia, heart palpitations and hallucinations.[104] The tranquillizers, antidepressants and other amphetamines used to treat hyperactivity had even worse side effects.[105] The strong sales of Ritalin and other hyperactivity drugs from the mid-1960s to the present day indicate that psychiatrists, as well as parents, were willing to overlook these shortcomings, chiefly because stimulants did what psychotherapy could not do: they calmed children down within minutes.

Another reason such side effects might have been tolerated is that biological psychiatrists were careful to describe their research in a cautiously optimistic fashion that left room for improvement. Ritalin might not cure hyperactivity and might cause troubling side effects, but with more research, its efficacy was expected to improve. An example of this attitude is found in the deceptively titled article, 'Psychopharmacology: The Picture Is Not Entirely Rosy'. Its author suggested that, while there was much work to be done, psychiatric ambitions of miracle pills would be realized eventually. What was required was continual research, optimism and faith in the ideology of biological psychiatry.[106] As the 1970s wore on, however, there were fewer reasons for such caution. For biological psychiatrists, the picture appeared to be very rosy indeed. In place of the psycho-analytical case studies that crowded journals during the 1950s and 1960s were the results of double-blind clinical trials of hyperactivity drugs, all of which appeared to indicate the efficacy of such drugs. One indication of this was that in 1976 Eveoleen Rexford was replaced by Melvin Lewis as the editor of the JAACP. Immediately, the journal shed its psychoanalytical trappings and became biologically oriented. Fittingly, the first article of the new era was Dennis P. Cantwell's 'Genetic Factors in the Hyperkinetic Syndrome'.

DSM-III, published in 1980, was also free of psychoanalytical and social psychiatric ideology and terminology.[107] Biological psychiatrist John S. Werry heralded this development as an indication that psychiatrists could once again take their place among their fellow doctors, considering themselves veritable neuroscientists.[108] In contrast, socially oriented psychiatrists Michael Rutter and David Shaffer acknowledged that the publication would be a scientific coming of age for psychiatry, but were not confident that this medi-calized approach was a good development. They argued that the manual now had a dogmatic style that could give false confidence to biological psychiatrists while alienating social workers and psychologists.[109] Hyperactivity was no longer hyperkinetic reaction of childhood, but Attention Deficit Disorder, so-called to reflect the prominence of attention deficits in hyperactive children; the dis-order would soon be renamed ADHD (in 1987), in recognition of the primacy of hyperactivity as a key symptom.[110] Instead of assessing an individual child and his or her environment and family situation, psychiatrists now had a checklist of symptoms to identify.

Despite the fact that four times the number of child disorders were included in DSM-III compared to DSM-II, hyperactivity, or ADD/ADHD, quickly proved to be the most common childhood psychiatric disorder in the manual. It was partly the dominance of the biological approach to hyperactivity that helped to make the disorder so popular. In eclipsing psychoanalytic and social psychiatric explanations for hyperactivity, biological psychiatry presented physicians and parents with a disorder that explained a great deal of problematic childhood behaviour, blamed it on a vague sort of

neurological malfunctioning and, crucially, supplied a pharmacological treatment that provided immediate results to most patients.
Such an approach was scientific, fitting psychiatry's desire to appear
medically authoritative, technological, in that it tapped into
psychopharmacological developments and ideology, and non-
judgemental, since it pinned the trouble not on dysfunctional
families, schools or societies, but rather on a glitch in the brain that
could be tweaked with stimulant drugs. Biological psychiatry's
answer to hyperactivity, the symbol of American educational shortcomings, might have been simple, but it was also effective.

It is interesting to imagine what Robert Felix would have
thought of it all. In 1964 he described an American psychiatric
profession that had fought for a generation to earn recognition and
respect from the medical community. Decrying the divisiveness of
his colleagues, he saw an opportunity for a 'warm, human, down to
earth' psychiatric profession that would be 'civilly active', 'serve the
community' and have both psychological and biological grounding.[111] In other words, he described a holistic, complementary and
comprehensive psychiatry that demanded the philosophical and
dynamic sophistication of psychoanalysis, the preventive and political action of social psychiatry and the technological and scientific
grounding of biological psychiatry. It is likely that if Felix's vision
of psychiatry had been realized, a far more nuanced, constructive
understanding of hyperactivity would have emerged.

Nearly half a century after Felix's remarks, psychiatry seems to
be at a similar crossroads. Mental illness is again seen to be one of
the most pernicious threats to health and governments are keen to
find prophylactic strategies. Although biological psychiatry remains
predominant, there are indications that social and quasi-psycho-
analytical or cognitive approaches to psychiatry are gathering
momentum. A number of studies have begun to question the efficacy of psychoactive drugs, claiming either that they act only as a
placebo or that their side effects may be more dangerous that the
symptoms they purport to treat. Other observers have suggested that
only '10% of current youthful users [of hyperactivity drugs] would
require medication if they had optimal family and school situations'.[112] In the UK, in the midst of draconian government cutbacks

at all levels, the government is keen to provide more funding for psychiatric counselling, especially for children seen to be at risk. According to Deputy Prime Minister Nick Clegg, the government's £400 million strategy 'means we can get these talking therapies to children before their problems become problems of a lifetime'.[113] Social psychiatry is also experiencing a renaissance under the banner, 'social determinants of mental health'. Dissatisfied with the biological approach to psychiatry and the disproportionate costs paid by society's poorest in terms of mental illness, a growing number of physicians and health policy makers, including David Satcher, the former surgeon general of the United States, are once again calling for preventive mental health strategies to dominate mental health policy. Perhaps this time, psychiatrists will think less of their professional interests and have the confidence to opt for a more pluralistic, sophisticated and, ultimately, more effective approach.

FOUR

Ritalin: Magic Bullet or Black Magic?

Introduction: What's in a Wonder Drug?

On one side of an advertisement found in the pages of a medical journal from the 1970s is an angry young boy, aged about ten, with light blonde hair, wearing basketball sneakers, jeans and a T-shirt. He has been playing with a Mini Makit set, a wooden construction toy, but has now torn apart the structure on which he has been working. Teeth clenched with eyes closed, he is pictured thrashing unhappily, gripping bits of his toy with both hands. His movement is such that the camera cannot keep up; the image is blurred, making the rods and discs of his Mini Makit set look the wings of an enormous flying insect in his tight little fists. On the other side of the page, the child is much calmer. Now he is still, quietly reading a book on the sofa. The book is somewhat obscured, but the image that is shown features medieval soldiers marching in a row, suggesting that it might be a children's history book. The boy looks like a completely different child; his face, relaxed now, is attractive, angelic even, in marked contrast to the scrunched-up, angry face that is on the opposite page. Despite his repose, it is clear that he is transfixed by his book, his slightly open mouth suggestive of his deep concentration. What can explain the drastic change in behaviour? A prescription for Ritalin.

The advertisement is remarkably detailed and clever. The 'before' picture portrays a boy who is playing with an educational toy, one designed to inspire creativity and engineering prowess. The fact that he has such a toy, combined with his clothes and haircut, indicate that he is from a middle-class family, and that his parents care about his education. His visceral frustration suggests that he knows what he wants to build with his Mini Makit set, but his inability to concentrate prevents him from doing so. The furious manner in which he rips the toy apart likely foreshadows a tremendous temper tantrum. That the boy's behaviour is uncontrollable even when he is playing at home makes one wonder how he could possibly behave in a school setting.

The boy in the 'after' picture, in contrast, has chosen not to play a game or run about at home, but instead quietly read a book. Looking closer, it appears that he has another book beside him, suggesting that, either he has become a voracious reader, or perhaps he is working intently on a homework project for history class. As the advertisement is aimed at physicians, a copious amount of text in small print surrounds the images that nonetheless dominate each page. The text does not explain the pictures in any way, but rather provides a psychiatric context through which the physician may interpret the scenes depicted. Above the 'before' picture, for example, there is a caption that states how children with minimal brain dysfunction may be 'aggressive, destructive, easily frustrated' and 'can't concentrate'. The caption beside the 'after' picture similarly adds medical meaning to the image, describing how 'it may be that stimulants act on higher (cortical) centers of the brain and thereby "stimulate" greater conscious awareness', thus suggesting that the boy's newfound academic abilities are due to the effects of Ritalin. Other bits of text highlight the efficacy of the drug and downplay the risk of side effects. For the general practitioner, paediatrician or psychiatrist confronted with a parent whose child's behaviour resembles that of the blonde boy in the 'before' picture, the advertisement is a compelling inducement to write out a prescription for Ritalin.

As described in the previous chapter, one of the most important factors in the rise of biological explanations for hyperactivity was the apparent efficacy of the stimulant drugs prescribed by biological psychiatrists to treat the disorder, most notably methylphenidate, which is better known by its trade name Ritalin. There have been many different drugs used to treat hyperactivity, including Dexedrine, Benzedrine, Cylert, Adderall, Strattera, Focalin and others, but Ritalin is the most emblematic and is the one that is the focus of this chapter. In many ways, Ritalin encapsulates the divisiveness of hyperactivity. While some physicians, parents and teachers see it as a magic bullet, calming children and helping them focus on their schoolwork, others see it as a dangerous tool of social control, stunting the natural growth and development of children and teaching them that psychoactive drugs are often a necessary condition of success and happiness. Depending on one's perspective, Ritalin represents all that is good about modern biomedicine and neurological approaches to psychiatry or the very opposite.

This chapter puts Ritalin under the microscope, and asks why the drug became such a popular and controversial treatment for hyperactivity. The quick response to this question, that it appeared to help hyperactive children, as advertisements for the drugs claim, is an important part of the answer, but does not completely address why Americans were willing to put their children on a powerful and possibly hazardous stimulant drug for a behavioural problem that could have been addressed in other ways. Many drugs have the desired effect in treating particular symptoms, but have been deemed unsuitable for widespread use for a variety of reasons. In some cases, they have dangerous side effects, which are seen to outweigh their benefits. A good example of this is thalidomide, which was prescribed to pregnant women between 1957 and 1961 to ameliorate morning sickness. Tragically, the drug was teratogenic, and caused fatalities and terrible birth defects in babies whose mothers had taken it. But although thalidomide was banned by most regulatory bodies in the early 1960s, it was soon found to have beneficial properties in other conditions, particularly cancers and autoimmune diseases. Its stigma, however, was such that it took until 1998 for thalidomide to be approved by the American Food and Drug Administration (FDA) for the treatment of leprosy, not a particularly widespread disease in the United States. The lingering memory of thalidomide's deformed victims will continue to hamper efforts to revive its use, despite its apparent potential as a 'wonder drug' for treating the symptoms of HIV/AIDS and myeloma.[1]

In other cases, the drug's purported benefits have not been enough to overcome its reputation as an illicit substance. Cannabis and opium were used in the nineteenth century to treat numerous conditions, but were ultimately criminalized, not because their therapeutic benefits were discredited, but rather because they became socially unacceptable.[2] While it could be said that morphine supplanted the medical use of opium, medical marijuana remains a contested treatment. Recently, the state of California has decided to crack down on medical marijuana dispensaries, despite the fact that they have been legal since the mid-1990s, because of the belief that many are simply fronts for drug dealing. Ironically, many pro-cannabis campaigners look to the past to find evidence to support the legalization of marijuana, for example, the Indian Hemp Drugs Commission report of 1893–4, which found that mild to moderate marijuana posed few risks to health.[3]

Possibly the most striking example of a potential wonder drug that failed to gain medical or social approval is dilysergic acid diethylamide, or LSD, which was being investigated around the time when Ritalin came onto the market in the 1950s. As historian Erika Dyck has described, psychiatrists Humphrey Osmond (1917–2004) and Abram Hoffer (1917–2009) began researching the therapeutic effects of the psychedelic drug in Weyburn, Saskatchewan in the early 1950s. They soon discovered that it had potential as a cure for alcoholism, which, much like hyperactivity, was increasingly being seen as a medical condition rather than a behavioural problem.[4] But, despite promising findings and initial support, especially within the province of Saskatchewan, the medical community was sceptical, in large part because it doubted Hoffer and Osmond's theoretical grounding, which combined social-psychological and medical models of addiction.[5] Even more damaging was the emerging 'acid panic', as LSD became the archetypal drug of 1960s counter-culture.[6] Although, like thalidomide, there has been renewed interest in the medical benefits of LSD, it will take a considerable shift in public opinion to resurrect LSD as a therapeutic, rather than a dangerous, drug.

If thalidomide, opium, cannabis and LSD failed to become acceptable treatments for conditions as serious as cancer, HIV/AIDS and alcoholism, why was Ritalin thought to be appropriate for use in hyperactive children? One might automatically retort that Ritalin has little in common with drugs such as these, but in contrast, Ritalin was also associated with criminal use, has numerous adverse effects, including some fatalities, and was the subject of considerable negative publicity, particularly after other amphetamines previously marketed as wonder drugs were targeted by regulatory authorities as being dangerous.[7] Most importantly, it was a drug aimed at children diagnosed with a controversial and contestable behavioural disorder, not alcoholism, cancer, leprosy or AIDS. It would appear that Ritalin had as many strikes against it becoming an approved and popular treatment as any of these other drugs, yet it is the one that became, at least to its advocates, a wonder drug. Why was this the case?

There are many explanations for Ritalin's popularity. Certainly the fact that many physicians, parents and patients believe that it is efficacious has been a major factor. But the ways in which Ritalin has fended off the various and continued criticisms of it suggest that its apparent effectiveness in correcting child behaviour tells only part of the story. Ritalin's resilience has also been buttressed by how aggressively its manufacturers, CIBA (1961–71), CIBA-Geigy (1971–96) and Novartis (1996–present), have marketed not only the drug as a treatment for hyperactivity but also the very notion of hyperactivity itself. In Ritalin, these companies had a best-selling drug that children were expected to take well into adulthood. As such, Ritalin helped to normalize the use of psychoactive drugs in children, thus enabling such young patients to become lifetime consumers of such medication. Ritalin also symbolized the notion that children's behavioural problems were not developmental, nor the fault of improper parenting, teaching or unhealthy environments, but a genetic, neurological malfunction. Ritalin's effectiveness in a young child not only made that child easier to manage but also suggested to parents that his/her neurological deficit was the primary, if not the only, factor to consider; if his/her behaviour deteriorated, then a higher dosage was required, rather than an examination of his/her social and educational surroundings. If he/she became depressed while on the drug, then an antidepressant was the solution, rather than analysing what was behind the depression or stopping the Ritalin prescription. Finally, as a brain booster that was

RITALIN: MAGIC BULLET OR BLACK MAGIC?

not only prescribed legitimately to hyperactive children, but used illicitly by students trying to get an academic edge, Ritalin raised a question similar to one asked by steroid users: if a drug can help a child (or adult) perform better academically, why not use it?

This chapter tells the story of Ritalin, from its origin as an antidepressant and 'pep' pill for elderly and depressed patients to its use in children, and describes the controversies that have continued to envelop the drug and its use. The history of Ritalin demonstrates that the debates that have surrounded the drug since its approval for use in children in 1961 have had less to do with whether or not it works and more with the philosophical and ideological issues inherent in deciding whether young children require psychoactive drugs to control their behaviour. As such, Ritalin highlights how parents, educators and physicians have wrestled with what constitutes a productive, happy and healthy childhood and whether childhood is a means to a more productive society or an end in itself.

From Energizing 'Oldsters' to Calming Children

The first time I saw an advertisement for Ritalin, I thought I was seeing things. Staring out at me from the pages of a 1966 volume of JAMA was not a wild-eyed, rambunctious child, but an elderly woman facing a mountain of potatoes to peel with a hang-dog face. The accompanying caption read: 'If chronic fatigue and mild depression make simple tasks seem this big . . . Ritalin relieves chronic fatigue that depresses and mild depression that fatigues'. Strangely, the picture on the facing page, which presumably was intended to demonstrate the restorative benefits of Ritalin, portrayed the woman looking only slightly less depressed. She did not appear to be as fatigued, and all of the potatoes had been peeled, but she stared blankly into the distance with an unidentifiable cooking implement in her hands. Despite the fact that she had been prescribed the drug to treat a condition that was as far removed from hyperactivity as possible, her blank, unfocused visage reminded me of the dull expressions of children I had taught who been prescribed Ritalin. As an advertisement, it has to be said that it is a failure (if I was a psychiatrist it certainly would not have convinced me to prescribe Ritalin to my fatigued and depressed patients), but it clearly indicates how Ritalin had a life before it became a hyperactivity drug for children.

Ritalin was first synthesized in 1944 by CIBA scientist Leandro Panizzon. Panizzon's wife, Marguerite, whose nickname was Rita, used the drug prior to playing tennis on account of her low blood pressure, and Panizzon named the stimulant after her.[8] The drug was patented in 1950 and then approved by the FDA for use in psychological disorders in 1955. Initially, Ritalin was used to treat drug-induced comas and to help patients recover from anaesthesia, but it was soon prescribed to treat other conditions, including depression, fatigue, senility, obesity, narcolepsy and schizophrenia, and to facilitate psychotherapy and electroshock therapy.[9] For those familiar with the work of historian Nicolas Rasmussen, this should not be too surprising. Amphetamines, such as Benzedrine, were used since the 1930s to combat a wide range of mental ailments.[10] In many cases, pharmaceutical companies had the drugs developed well before they identified the disorders the drugs were meant to alleviate. Likewise, in the case of Ritalin, CIBA's marketing department had a wide range of patients in mind. Although the advertisement featuring the elderly woman and her potatoes was obviously aimed at outpatients, CIBA also targeted institutionalized patients. A 1956 advertisement, for example, featured a woman dressed in hospital garb cowering in the corner of a bare room near a radiator. As the advertisement described, Ritalin could bring hospitalized patients such as these 'out of the corner' and was said to be 'effective in awaking patients to reality, even in "severe deteriorated schizophrenia of long standing"'. The drug helped to make 'such patients more amenable to therapy, suggestion, and social participation'. As sociologist Ilina Singh suggests, and most Ritalin adverts from the period indicate, CIBA targeted both male and female middle-aged and elderly patients suffering from a number of mild, moderate and severe afflictions.[11] Similarly, a number of medical articles from the late 1950s indicated that the drug was geared towards treating 'oldsters', 'troublesome, miserable old people' for whom a strong cup of coffee was not enough.[12] Later advertisements, however, tended to focus on housewives, such as the woman with the potatoes, who were suffering from the vaguely medical 'tired housewife syndrome'.[13]

The fact that Ritalin was first marketed to patients who were about as far removed as possible in terms of age and symptoms from hyperactive children is instructive in a number of ways. It demonstrates how many psychoactive drugs during the first wave of psychopharmacology during the 1950s were developed without a clear patient group or set of symptoms in mind. Just as Charles Bradley stumbled into discovering that amphetamines could help schoolchildren focus academically while trying to ease their pneumoencephalography-induced headaches during the 1930s, it was not unusual for psychoactive drugs to take a convoluted path towards an application that was both clinically and financially beneficial. Chlorpromazine, the first antipsychotic, for example, had its roots in nineteenth-century German coal-tar chemistry, and was derived from antihistamines whose anti-microbial properties were also being explored.[14] Serendipity, chance and luck had considerable roles to play in finding a clinical home for newly developed drugs and, in many cases, 'the cure preceded the ailment'.[15]

The lengths CIBA went to in order to find a market for Ritalin also demonstrated the financial pressure to find clinical uses for drugs developed in research. CIBA's efforts to market Ritalin for conditions ranging from obesity and narcolepsy to depression and hyperactivity did not necessarily indicate a desperation to find an application for its patented product, but certainly demonstrate an aggressive approach.[16] Behind the advertisements would be the countless trips to hospitals, clinics and practices made by 'detail men', CIBA's sales representatives.[17] As historian Nancy Tomes has described:

> under the American patent system, drug companies had roughly twenty years to profit from a new prescription drug; to build market share in a brutally competitive industry, they had a strong incentive to court physicians aggressively.[18]

Historian Nathan Moon has also emphasized CIBA's ability to exploit multiple markets for the application of Ritalin. While Moon sees this as evidence of CIBA's receptivity to the needs of psychiatrists, it is also important to note the financial imperative the company faced in finding a market for their product.[19]

Ironically, the chief competitor CIBA faced in tapping into the market of mildly depressed older patients was not necessarily one of the other antidepressant drugs being developed, but another stimulant: caffeine. Ritalin was often marketed as being 'less potent than amphetamine but more so than caffeine'.[20] While the amount of coffee or tea required to equal a typical dose of Ritalin might have been impractical from a pharmacological standpoint, the social and emotional benefits of a 'nice cup of tea' shared with friends should not be underestimated either. Just as Ritalin's efficacy in treating mildly depressed elderly patients are now being investigated again, many studies have demonstrated the numerous benefits of serving generous amounts of coffee and tea in geriatric and Alzheimer's patients.[21] Caffeine also had potential as a treatment for hyperactive children, as is discussed below.

Perhaps to get around the fact that commonly consumed beverages could have a similar effect as their drug, CIBA not only advertised Ritalin as an effective pep pill, but also marketed the very idea that mild depression was a ubiquitous pathology in middle-aged and elderly people. That Ritalin could be used to treat patients ranging from institutionalized schizophrenics to fatigued 'oldsters' also foreshadowed the applicability of the drug in children with a wide range of behavioural problems. Ritalin could be used in quite disturbed children, but also children who had mild symptoms; the only difference would be the dose prescribed. CIBA's targeting of mildly depressed and fatigued elderly people, particularly tired housewives, individuals who might have benefited from more companionship, social engagement and physical activity, is also oddly reminiscent of its marketing of the notion of hyperactivity which in essence pathologized childhood behaviours that might otherwise be considered quite normal in most children. In both cases, concern about the troublesome behaviours presented by both old and young patients was also exaggerated by demographic factors; just as psychiatrists were worried about their ability to treat all the mentally disturbed Baby Boomers, post-war increases in life expectancy meant that physicians had to adapt to the 'difficult mental and physical adjustments accompanying old age'.[22] Despite the many differences inherent in depressed 'oldsters' and hyperactive children, therefore, there are also many connections between them, their perceived disorders and the drug believed to help them. Perhaps most profound is that in each case, represented by the elderly woman and her potatoes and the hyperactive boys depicted bouncing around in subsequent advertisements, we can see that something is the matter, but we might well wonder whether a stimulant drug is an effective or ethical solution in either.

'Drugs That Help Control the Unruly Child'

Ritalin only had limited success as an antidepressant during the 1950s and 1960s, despite CIBA's efforts to market the drug to the mildly depressed middle-aged and elderly. It is difficult to explain why, particularly since many contemporary observers believed that the drug was effective and given recent efforts to re-brand the drug as an antidepressant for geriatric patients.[23] It is possible that CIBA's decision to continue advertising the antidepressive qualities of Ritalin after it was approved for use in hyperactivity in 1961 bemused some physicians, not to mention their patients. Strange though it may sound, there must have been many families during the 1960s in which a grandmother was taking Ritalin to pick her up while her grandson was taking the same drug to calm him down. It is also likely that mildly depressed patients simply preferred the tranquillizing effects of best-sellers such as Miltown and Valium, rather than the stimulation of Ritalin, particularly if there was something other than neurology underlying their symptoms.

Despite CIBA's efforts to market Ritalin as an antidepressant, it is certainly best known as a treatment for hyperactivity. As mentioned in chapter One, Charles Bradley serendipitously discovered that amphetamines, specifically Benzedrine, could help children at his psychiatric institution focus and perform better academically. Although hyperactivity experts and many historians continually point to Bradley's use of amphetamines during the 1930s to contend that there was a tradition of using stimulants to treat behavioural problems, it took 25 years for the Rhode Island psychiatrist's discovery to be replicated and applied to hyperactivity.[24] There were isolated cases of employing stimulants to treat behavioural problems, but no controlled studies were undertaken until the 1960s.[25] The fact that Ritalin was not marketed as a hyperactivity treatment until 1961, seventeen years after it was synthesized, is further evidence that there was little interest in prescribing stimulants to disturbed children until the launch of Sputnik and the crisis in education it fomented. Or, as sociologist Peter Conrad has observed, the 'treatment was available long before the disorder treated was clearly conceptualized'.[26]

Indeed, the primary reason why stimulants were not employed to treat hyperactivity prior to the late 1950s was that hyperactive children were simply not seen as a major medical concern before that point. But there were other reasons why their use was limited until the late 1950s. The apparently paradoxical effect that stimulants such as Ritalin had on hyperactive children, for example, presented a puzzle for many physicians. It did not make intuitive sense to prescribe a stimulant to a child who needed to settle down, rather than perk up. In fact, one of the first studies to explore the use of Ritalin in children's behavioural problems suggested that hyperactivity itself was a side effect of the drug.[27] Although recent research suggests that Ritalin's function in elevating norepinephrine levels helps to explain the paradox, physicians have long expressed bewilderment at the stimulant's soothing influence.[28]

Despite its paradoxical action, Ritalin was being explored for use in hyperactive children as early as the late 1950s. One of the earliest clinical trials conducted was done in 1959 by Kansas City psychiatrists George Lytton and Mauricio Knobel, who found that the drug improved the behaviour of the twenty children they tested.[29] Four years later a much larger, controlled trial of the drug was conducted by psychiatrist Leon Eisenberg and C. Keith Conners. Eisenberg had been involved in earlier studies that investigated the effectiveness of psychoactive drugs in hyperactive children, particularly in comparison to psychotherapy. Not believing that psychotherapy was suitable for such children, and going as far as to suggest that many psychoanalysts refused to take on hyperactive patients because of this, Eisenberg believed that drugs could be an alterna-tive.[30] Funded by NIMH, Eisenberg and Conners's tests are thought to be the first to demonstrate Ritalin's efficacy in treating disturbed children and were largely responsible for convincing physicians that stimulants could calm down hyperactive children and help them focus.[31] A close look at their findings, however, reveals that the re-searchers were more cautious about Ritalin than would be expected in such a landmark study, and that their results did not amount to an endorsement of the use of Ritalin in a large percentage of Ameri-can children.

First, Eisenberg and Conners's test subjects were residential care patients, not schoolchildren, which suggests that they were suffering from quite severe behavioural symptoms.[32] One of their previous studies had focused on delinquent children at a training school, again indicating that the researchers were concerned with fairly disturbed and troubled children.[33] Second, the drug appeared to be more effective in children of lower intelligence than those of higher intelligence.[34] This is also somewhat surprising in retrospect, considering that hyperactivity is often seen as a disorder that prevents children of average or high intelligence from reaching their potential. Third, the authors found that Ritalin's effects were substantial, but also somewhat alarming, since 70 per cent of their subjects in the drug group suffered side effects, some significant enough to put the double-blind aspect of the study at risk and thus raise the potential for bias.[35] Again, this is interesting, since one of the reasons Ritalin was considered for use in hyperactive children was that it was thought to have fewer and less severe side effects than other substances, including other stimulants.[36] In conclusion, Eisenberg and Conners believed that Ritalin showed promise, but refrained from giving the drug a blanket endorsement given the wide variance in degree and manner of the changes it appeared to cause. The authors urged that further study be done on the drug, including its effects on the personality of its users.[37]

Despite the caution inherent in their conclusions, Eisenberg and Conners's study was seen to provide incontrovertible evidence that Ritalin was beneficial to hyperactive children. In a more subtle way, the study also signified a shift in the way in which prospective therapies for children would be studied and reported. As commentator Joel Zrull described, Eisenberg and Conners's study was an example of a new approach with respect to the 'methods of assessing the effects of drugs on human behavior (and in this case the behavior of children)'.[38] Instead of clinical evaluations, typically done in a doctor's office, the 'everyday' behaviour of patients would be assessed in the form of double-blind studies. Although the thalidomide tragedy and subsequent government hearings into ensuring the safety of new drugs also played a major role in, and provided good reason for, this epistemological shift, it is possible that the humanity, idiosyncrasies and individuality of specific patients, particularly psychiatric patients, was lost to a degree in the privileging of quantifiable evidence from randomly controlled trials versus anecdotal and qualitative clinical evidence. The more physicians took their lead from the results of double-blind trials, not to mention the marketing of pharmaceutical companies, the more they saw their patients as anonymous subjects, rather than unique individuals enveloped in complex personal, familial and social circumstances. Apart from Ritalin's efficacy, the marketing of pharmaceutical companies and the desires of parents, it is perhaps this shift that is most important in explaining the success of Ritalin.

Following Eisenberg and Conners's trials and those that followed, it did not take long for Ritalin to be triumphed not only in medical journals, but also in the media. According to a 1970 article in the *New York Times*, Ritalin was the drug that could 'help to control the unruly child'.[39] In the article, which focused on Rhode Island, the birthplace of stimulant drug therapy for children, the story of the archetypal 'Billy the Wall Climber' was told:

> Every teacher knows Billy the Wall Climber. He's got so much energy that he cannot sit still long enough to add 2 and 2. He's throwing paper clips at the boy across the aisle, shoving on the lunch line, fighting and stealing in the schoolyard. In days past, he might have spent much of his time dunking some little girl's pigtails into the inkwell. He never does learn to read well, and often drops out of school into delinquency, even though tests show he has adequate

or even superior intelligence. Until recently, he could get little help and was, in effect, written off by many teachers and schools.[40]

The story proceeded to describe how these 'wall-climbers' were now treated with stimulants, which 'had a strange effect on these hyperactive youngsters', calming them down and helping them concentrate better on their schoolwork.[41] Maurice Laufer and Leon Eisenberg were also quoted, enthusing about how Ritalin could benefit children with behaviour problems.

Another article centred on the story of 'Jackie D', a six-year-old 'with big brown eyes' who 'was so bad that his mother was at her wit's end'. Similarly to Billy the Wall Climber, Jackie

could not sit still, he fought with all the other children on the block, was so clumsy that he could not ride a bicycle, had trouble reading and got so frustrated with his first-grade arithmetic that he would tear up his lessons.[42]

Once Jackie began taking Ritalin, however, he transformed from his 'usual self' into a 'quiet, coordinated' boy who did 'well enough in his lessons to be promoted to second grade'.[43] Jackie was described as 'one of countless thousands of American youngsters with normal or even high intelligence who get Ritalin', a remedy referred to as 'black magic when it works', 'the penicillin of children with learning disabilities' and 'as effective as insulin in diabetes' in 'appropriately selected patients'.[44] As the article indicated that anywhere between 5 and 20 per cent of American children were thought to suffer from hyperactivity, the 'countless thousands' were expected to become many millions.[45]

Such success stories also detailed the controversial side of Ritalin. The mechanism of the drug was unclear, as one journalist explained, and many children reported side effects, such as insomnia and loss of appetite.[46] Although psychiatrists such as Eisenberg stressed, after following up on Charles Bradley's patients during the 1930s, that long-term use was not thought to cause addiction or emotional damage, other experts were concerned about the unintended consequences of extended use. As Richard Young, a psychology professor at Indiana University, exclaimed:

> I shudder when I hear my colleagues suggest you can go ahead and give drugs to children to see what their behavior are [sic] like . . . We really don't know what are the effects of a lot of these drugs on a lot of processes over the long run.[47]

In reply, Sidney Adler, a California paediatrician, argued that:

> I don't know what the drug will do in 20 years . . . but I have to try to do what we can do now to keep the kid from winding up in juvenile hall.[48]

Instead of advocating caution, Adler expressed admiration for a 'practical, gutsy' colleague from the 'boondocks' who reported that Ritalin had helped one of his rural patients progress from failing consistently in school to achieving 'straight A marks'.[49] Given the fears about epidemic rates of childhood mental disorder, it is not particularly surprising that some physicians saw the prescription of Ritalin as not morally questionable, but as an example of heroic medical treatment.

Nevertheless, there were many other concerns about the drug. Its association with illicit amphetamines, known vernacularly as speed, bennies, uppers, crank or crystal, was particularly damaging, and contributed to the banning of Ritalin in Sweden during the late 1960s.[50] With the legal production of amphetamines topping ten billion tablets per year, their medical use was also cause for concern.[51] In response, the FDA and a panel of the National Academy of Sciences, known as the 'Task Force on Drug Abuse' recommended to a Senate subcommittee in 1971 that the potential for Ritalin abuse was such that it should be placed 'in the same strictly controlled classification as morphine and other valuable but dangerous drugs'.[52] The subcommittee was told that Ritalin had led to a prominent drug abuse problem in many cities, particularly Seattle where it was described as the 'No. 1 drug abuse problem', causing multiple health problems, including heart disease.[53] Instead of taking it orally as prescribed, abusers dissolved Ritalin and then injected it.[54] Although Ritalin abuse by adults was emphasized there were other reports of 'children swapping their pills in the school yard with unfortunate effects'.[55]

CIBA-Geigy, then the manufacturer of Ritalin, responded to the Senate subcommittee that they knew of no evidence documenting the abuse of their product and that reclassification would stigmatize the drug. Despite the company's protestations, the Task Force on Drug Abuse also warned that legitimate use of Ritalin was also excessive and that physicians were prescribing it to children 'without adequate diagnostic qualification'. Such concerns reflect the fact that some physicians actually employed Ritalin as a diagnostic tool; the drug's efficacy distinguished the 'pure' hyperactive child from children whose disruptiveness was purposeful and indicative of antisocial behaviour.[56] They also drew attention to the corporation's muscular marketing of Ritalin. As one observer noted in the early 1970s, 'CIBA advertises ad nauseam, in medical magazine spreads running to seven full pages for Ritalin'.[57] Others claimed that the 'drug industry has continued to promote the use of amphetamines for disturbed children and is largely responsible for extending the practice'.[58] In a story for the *Village Voice*, it was reported how, in a 1971 sales report, a CIBA executive encouraged his salesmen to become 'more effective pushers' by using 'ingenuity'.[59] Highlighted in the report were an anonymous salesman in Paducah, Kentucky, who established a screening programme for preschool children to identify those likely to have learning disabilities, and a representative in South Bend, Indiana, who organized a meeting of special educators where a physician demonstrated the effectiveness of Ritalin using two of his hyperactive patients. Another CIBA employee stressed looking beyond education professionals, specifically urging his colleagues to concentrate on juvenile court officers and probation officers. As the executive enthused: 'That's getting involvement, folks.'[60]

Early hyperactivity critics Peter Schrag and Diane Divoky also highlighted the lengths to which CIBA went to market their product and the idea of hyperactivity. According to the California authors, it was 'nearly impossible to overestimate the role of the pharmaceutical houses in shaping medical and lay opinion about learning-disabled children'.[61] CIBA not only funded studies into stimulant therapy conducted by Conners, Leon Oettinger and others, it also paid such 'authorities' to present their findings at meetings for organizations such as the Association for Children with Learning Difficulties. According to Oettinger, CIBA's generosity was such that: 'Whenever we need money . . . they give us some more'.[62] Although the extent of the relationship, and the money exchanged, between CIBA and researchers such as Oettinger was unclear, there was little doubt that a symbiotic relationship existed between the two parties.

Schrag and Divoky were also concerned about CIBA's

> aggressive promotion and sales campaign pushing not only the drug but the ailments it is supposed to mitigate, if not to cure, a brilliant blend of social mythology about bright happy classrooms with bright happy children and carefully selected citations from the medical literature which, on closer inspection, totally fail to support the conclusions that the advertising suggests.[63]

CIBA's sales campaign not only included advertising, but also publications, such as *The MBD Child: A Guide for Parents* and the *Physician's Handbook: Screening for MBD* (MBD being Minimal Brain Dysfunction/ Damage), as well as organizing community and PTA meetings to promote both hyperactivity and CIBA's remedy.[64] The pharmaceutical company also produced a film, entitled *The Hyperactive Child*, which they distributed widely and showed at such meetings. Although the FDA ordered CIBA and other pharmaceutical companies to stop marketing directly to parents and teachers, Schrag and Divoky believed it did little to affect the sales of Ritalin, which by the early 1970s dominated 80 per cent of the hyperactivity market, despite the fact that it was more expensive than similar products, such as Dexedrine.[65]

Ritalin's side effects were also cause for concern. Among those reported were insomnia, depression, anorexia, bed-wetting, irritability, cardiovascular problems and hallucinations; parents and physicians also worried about the long-term use of the drug. In one case reported in *Life* magazine, the drug appeared to exacerbate one patient's disturbing behaviour. 'Mike' had trouble reading, required counselling, could not cope in regular school, where he was teased 'mercilessly', and engaged in 'foul and violent' behaviour at home, directed especially at his younger sister. He threatened to commit suicide and was thought to be headed for institutionalization. As 'a last resort' his physician took him off Ritalin and, within 24 hours, Mike's behaviour had improved, much to the doctor's surprise.[66] In a different case, the drug appeared to calm down a schoolgirl too much:

> The school called and said she was . . . like a zombie . . . She used to have a high vocabulary and was very social. On it [Ritalin] she sat in a corner, sucked her thumb, wouldn't talk at all.[67]

Although Ritalin was seen to have fewer side effects than dextroamphetamine or chlorpromazine in a 1971 study, the ones it did have in two of the 25 subjects were nevertheless alarming. After taking 10 mg of Ritalin, one 30-month-old child 'screamed for several hours until he fell asleep, exhausted'.[68] Another child, six years old,

> who had no previous signs of psychosis and who was well adjusted . . . was described as being 'in a world of his own and agitated'. On the second day he developed visual and tactile hallucinations, saying that he 'saw and felt worms all over him'. He became more agitated and acted in a bizarre way. On the third day, when no medica- [sic] was given, he returned to normal.[69]

Other less striking side effects seen in this study included stomach aches, anorexia, irritability, sadness, bed-wetting, nail-biting, 'looking dazed' and facial tics. Despite these side effects, the researchers, who were also clinicians, declared that Ritalin had became their 'drug of choice' for this group of hyperactive children.[70]

It is worth mentioning that some of the members of this specific 1971 study team would become influential advocates of child psychopharmacology. More outspoken Ritalin advocates, such as Leon Oettinger, also tended to downplay the danger of the drug's side effects, or suggested combination drug therapy to quell them.[71] In contrast, other physicians were considerably more alarmed about Ritalin's side effects and recommended more research, particularly on their long-term cardiovascular and anorexic effects, and their effects on younger children.[72] Concern about side effects also moved many parents to remove their children from controlled trials of Ritalin and other stimulant drugs.[73] Taking 'drug holidays', which consisted of reducing a child's dosage during the summer or Christmas holidays, was often recommended by some as a way of reducing adverse effects, but others warned that this could reduce the efficacy of the drug once dosage levels returned to normal.[74] Seeking an alternative stimulant that might have fewer side effects, a number of researchers during the 1970s considered the efficacy of caffeine in treating hyperactive children. One of the first to do so, Robert Schnackenberg, got the idea from his patients, who self-medicated with coffee. Schnackenberg argued that caffeine not only had fewer side effects, it was also cheaper and less controversial. He proceeded to claim that while children in North America did not tend to drink caffeinated beverages, those in Latin America did, and this helped to explain why hyperactivity was rare in South America.[75]

Although it is more likely that cultural differences between South and North America were more important than rates of child caffeine consumption in explaining such discrepancies (Latin American rates of hyperactivity are also now on a par with those in North America, according to some studies), I also experienced cases of young people self-medicating with caffeinated beverages while working as a youth counsellor during the late 1990s.[76] In one instance, a young man took a two-litre bottle of Pepsi Cola with him everywhere in case he needed a 'fix'. Although he did not want to take Ritalin, his physician urged him to do so to reduce the amount of sugar, calories and chemicals he was consuming by self-medicating. Another youth would consume a one-litre pot of coffee every morning when he awoke. Impatient for this to brew, he would drink a cup of instant coffee while he waited.

Although Schnackenberg found caffeine to be effective, others did not. A 1975 comparison of caffeine and methylphenidate explained that physicians might well be inclined to prescribe caffeine in order to avoid the side effects of Ritalin, but that when compared head to head, Ritalin was more effective.[77] Others similarly declared that caffeine was not a viable alternative, despite the positive findings of Schnackenberg and others.[78] Given Ritalin's adverse effects, its manufacturer's questionable marketing efforts, its association with illegal amphetamines and the fact that it simply did not work for many children, it is a testament to the drug's resilience that caffeine did not emerge as a serious rival.

Perhaps more damaging to Ritalin's image than these factors, however, was its own popularity. While it was believed that between 200,000 and 300,000 children were being prescribed hyperactivity drugs by the early 1970s, NIMH reported that up to 4,000,000 hyperactive children could also benefit from such medication.[79] A 1970 story in the *Washington Post*, which revealed that up to 10 per cent of schoolchildren in Omaha, Nebraska were being prescribed behaviour-modifying drugs such as Ritalin, put a spotlight on such concerns and spurred Congressional hearings into the issue.[80] Although problems with the Omaha data emerged, concerns were also raised about the widespread use of hyperactivity drugs in California, Michigan and Minnesota, where it was claimed that African American students in Minneapolis were being especially singled out for drug treatment.[81] Fears about the 'excessive reliance on medication as the "treatment of choice"' in cases of hyperactivity centred not only on the drug's short- and long-term physical effects, but also the broader impact of relying on such medications to change behaviour.[82] As one group of researchers warned, psychoactive drugs eroded the ability of groups and individuals to 'make provisions and develop strategies of human relatedness, which serve to regulate . . . anxiety, grief, rage and more extreme forms of behavior'.[83] In other words, such drugs acted as a crutch, preventing children from developing their own strategies to cope with their academic and behavioural shortcomings. To University of Iowa child psychiatrist Mark Stewart, children relying on Ritalin would have difficulty determining what their 'undrugged personality' was, as would their parents.[84]

Concerns about the overuse of Ritalin were directly associated with the fluidity and applicability of hyperactivity as a diagnosis, or as one observer noted, 'lack of conceptual clarity, combined with unbridled enthusiasm, has produced almost total chaos'.[85] A prominent Canadian psychiatrist, for instance, observed that 'pediatricians and teachers in a good-sized Canadian city reached virtually no agreement on any symptom of hyperactivity'.[86] This led to the danger of 'potentially overprescribing stimulants to a vast segment of the population'.[87] A special educator in Muncie, Indiana echoed such contentions, declaring that 'if a child got through our screens without something being picked up, we'd call him Jesus Christ'.[88] A report in *Time* similarly stated that it was 'far too easy for a teacher to mistake normal childhood restlessness for hyperkinesis or some other ailment requiring treatment by drugs'. A psychologist cited in the same article suggested that part of the problem was that the symptoms of hyperactivity represented 'almost everything that adults don't like about children'.[89] Others took a similarly contrarian perspective, arguing that 'these children described as suffering from hyperactivity are in fact suffering from what may be called Holt's complaint, the main symptom of which is an inability to stomach American education'.[90] As more children were diagnosed with hyperactivity and prescribed Ritalin, debates about the drug and the disorder it was meant to treat grew louder and more polemical.

The diagnostic parameters for hyperactivity diagnoses were clarified somewhat with the publication of DSM-III and the emergence of the term ADD, although the temporary removal of the word 'hyperactivity' from the term added another element of confusion and uncertainty. But hyperactivity remained a diagnostic category that was seemingly applied with ease. Media stories suggested that parents were often pressured by school or medical authorities into allowing their children to be prescribed Ritalin.[91] One mother was told that her son did not really need Ritalin, but her physicians suggested to her that 'to please the school, why don't you give him them anyway?'[92] In other cases, as historian Nicolas Rasmussen has described, the pressure to prescribe emanated from parents who aggressively demanded prescriptions for their children, increasingly so during the 1980s.[93] Even a few proponents of drug therapy for hyperactive children, such as Eric Denhoff, estimated that as many as half of the children prescribed stimulants in his state of Rhode Island should not have been.[94] Others warned that many physicians failed to recognize that medication was only one aspect of a broader treatment regimen that should also include behavioural modification, counselling, educational strategies and ample consideration of the child's domestic, academic and social environment.[95] To many observers, Ritalin 'was the first approach advised' when it should have been 'the last resort considered'.[96]

Despite all the problems associated with, and concerns about, Ritalin, the use of the drug continued to escalate throughout the 1970s, 1980s and 1990s. Whereas it was estimated that between 300,000 and 500,000 children were being prescribed stimulants for hyperactivity in 1980, in 1987 the number was 750,000 and rates rose to 1,800,000 in 1993 and 2,600,000 in 1995.[97] Such increases could be expected since diagnoses of hyperactivity were also escalating during this period, but this does not completely explain why Ritalin and other psychoactive drugs became the predominant treatment for hyperactivity, despite the presence of alternative therapies. Why, in the face of so many concerns, did Ritalin become so popular?

The simple answer, as mentioned above, was the perception that it worked. But what does that phrase, 'it worked', actually mean? When the phrase is unpacked, it becomes clearer that the efficacy of Ritalin involved more than simply alleviating the symptoms of hyperactivity. For psychiatrists, often used to dealing with intractable, difficult cases, such drugs offered the sort of clinical successes that were enjoyed by most physicians on a regular basis. As hyperactivity pioneer Maurice Laufer described, Ritalin created 'one of the few situations in which you can do something quickly for people'.[98] Rather than engaging in months or years of counselling, or delving into a patient's social and educational history, Ritalin gave psychiatrists a degree of instant gratification. For one physician it was 'fascinating and exciting to watch a child who awakes mean and irritable. Within 15 to 30 minutes after taking methylphenidate he becomes calm and cooperative and is able to sustain concentration for four hours.'[99] Although the marketing of such drugs by the pharmaceutical industry and psychiatry's desire to be seen as scientifically sophisticated certainly also played a role in making Ritalin ubiquitous, the drug's ability to generate a positive clinical encounter for patient, parent and psychiatrist should not be underestimated.

Psychiatrists might have had reservations about prescribing powerful stimulants to children, but when balanced against the dire prospects projected for hyperactive children who were untreated, the willingness to do so also becomes more understandable. For psychiatrist James Swanson, medication could 'mean the difference between a kid ending up at Berkeley and ending up in prison'.[100] Paediatrician Sidney Adler added:

> If we could figure out how to turn kids on in a more mean-ingful way, then I would be the first to say 'Throw out the drugs!' But we have to use them as tools to help these kids from going down the drain.[101]

Adler's focus on using Ritalin as a tool is also indicative. Ritalin was often seen as the pathway towards the sort of effective relationships and positive life experiences that would engender confidence and healthy self-esteem and prevent the psychological problems also associated with hyperactivity. As Laufer suggested, 'if you get to the child early, before the secondary emotional problems set in . . . this is all they need'.[102] When viewed from this perspective, the decision to prescribe Ritalin becomes less about eliminating behaviours that annoy teachers and parents and more about preventing future mental health problems.

Parents also saw Ritalin as being more than medication. The drug offered parents the prospect of reaching 'the good kid' hidden beneath the layers of disruptive behaviour.[103] One mother featured in a *Time* magazine article entitled 'Those Mean Little Kids' described her difficulties managing her son:

> I don't know what's the matter – I just can't handle him. He won't do anything I tell him. He won't sit still for a minute, he smashes things, he's mean to his brothers and sisters,

and when he wants something and I don't give it to him right away, he throws a temper tantrum.[104]

After he was on Ritalin she declared: 'Now I can love this child again.' The contented smile of a mother embracing her child in a Ritalin advertisement from the 1970s suggested that Ritalin could patch the damage done by hyperactivity to the relationship between mother and child. Such sentiments were common among mothers whose children had been prescribed the drug, many of whom might have resorted to tranquillizers and other drugs to treat their own mental health problems.[105] It is likely that the drug was also preferable to corporal punishment, which was becoming less acceptable as Ritalin became more popular.[106] Ritalin promised redemption for children whose behavioural problems prevented them from reaching their potential, for parents who were blamed for their child's hyperactivity and even for teachers whose instructional inadequacies were often singled out as a contributing factor. Perhaps most importantly, Ritalin offered what other magic bullets provided; it offered hope.

During the 2000s the gulf between Ritalin's advocates and detractors widened even more. While the drug's usage became increasingly commonplace and even normalized, the emergence of the Internet meant that dissenting opinions could easily find an outlet and an audience. On one end of the spectrum of debate were those who believed that, if Ritalin helped individuals diagnosed with hyperactivity succeed academically, perhaps the drug's benefits could be enjoyed by all. Such opinions were expressed cogently in the first issue of the *American Journal of Bioethics: Neuroscience*, where sociologist Ilina Singh and paediatrician Kelly Kelleher discussed 'Neuroenhancement in Young People'. The authors explained that since young people were using stimulant drugs illicitly to give them an academic edge, and since such medications 'from an ethical perspective' were no different from 'non-drug strategies widely used', such as vitamins, brain exercises and early music learning, drugs such as Ritalin should be more easily accessible.[107] Although the authors delineated the ethical and practical implications of such a change in health policy, they also argued that 'all young people ought to have equal access to existing resources to improve themselves and their performance'.[108] Neuroenhancement through drugs such as Ritalin was presented as not only inevitable, but also a tool for distributive justice.

On the other end of the spectrum were those who believed that the adverse effects of Ritalin and other hyperactivity drugs suggested that their use should be restricted, if not banned altogether. Such concerns emerged during the late 1990s and 2000s, when a series of reports emerged about the effects of such drugs on the cardiovascular system, spurring the American Heart Foundation to issue guidelines about their use in children.[109] One well-publicized case, for example, was that of Matthew Smith, a fourteen-year-old whose fatal heart failure was attributed to long-term Ritalin use.[110] Guidelines were not enough for Smith's parents, who urged parents to take their children off the drug and advocated alternative approaches to hyperactivity.[111]

Although the number of children believed to be at risk was low, a series of deaths related to hyperactivity drug Adderall prompted Health Canada to ban it temporarily in 2005.[112] The American FDA did not follow suit, but an FDA advisory committee recommended in 2006 that guidelines and warnings be strengthened to reflect such risks. Steven E. Nissen, a consultant for the advisory committee, believed that the risk of serious cardiovascular problems 'warranted strong and immediate action' and argued that hyperactivity drugs be subject to 'more selective and restricted use'.[113] In response, the FDA 'directed the manufacturers of all ADHD medicines to add a "black box" warning to their products, pointing to the potential cardiovascular risks'.[114]

Such measures did not put an end to the debate. Paediatrician Matthew Knight countered that the risk of stimulant death was outweighed by the benefits of such drugs.[115] A quartet of physicians similarly contended in *Pediatrics* that the risk of cardiovascular failure in children on Ritalin was no different from those in the general population.[116] A letter in response to the article, however, replied that although the nineteen fatalities related to hyperactivity medication that had been reported to the FDA was not a large number, it likely represented between 1 and 10 per cent of the actual figure. The letter writer also questioned the motives of the article's authors; all of them reportedly received funding from pharmaceutical companies.[117]

Somewhere in between the enormous gulf that exists between those who would like Ritalin to become a readily accessible brain booster and those who want it abolished lies a more sensible approach to the drug and the disorder it alleviates. The history of Ritalin demonstrates that there are many aspects to consider in determining whether it is a magic bullet or black magic. Ultimately, it is neither. Ritalin and the concept of hyperactivity may have been marketed aggressively by CIBA and its successors, but the history of Sputnik and the resulting American educational crisis suggests that the company was responding to, in addition to creating, a demand. The failure of Ritalin as a 'pep pill' for geriatrics, despite a similarly assertive marketing campaign, highlights how advertising can only do so much to manufacture an epidemic. Ritalin may have been chemically similar to illicit amphetamines and stimulants, such as speed and cocaine, but it was also not too far removed from caffeine. It certainly had side effects, but if it had the potential to put troubled children back on the right track, repairing damaged familial relationships in the process, it is somewhat understandable that parents, teachers and physicians accepted such risks. Seeing Ritalin as either magic bullet or black magic is a simplistic assessment of what is a highly complex emotive and ethical issue.

This being the case, is it enough for historians to sit on the fence and blithely pronounce that there are two sides to every story? Certainly not. The history of Ritalin is complicated, but there are lessons hidden among the ideology and rhetoric that dominate the debates. Ritalin 'worked' as a treatment for hyperactivity to the extent that it reduced the symptoms of 80 per cent of the hyperactive children who took it, but this is not the same thing as saying that it helped those children.[118] Likewise, answering why the drug became so popular is not the same thing as determining whether or not it should be prescribed. Given the amount of clinical and anecdotal evidence available, it would be difficult to argue that Ritalin does not have the potential to help at least some children. But it also has the potential to harm them, not simply by its adverse effects, but also by shifting attention from all the other aspects of a child's life that have bearing on his or her behaviour. Ritalin teaches children, and their parents, teachers and physicians, to turn to chemical solutions for problems that transcend the merely neurological. It is too facile and mechanical an answer for problems that are complicated and multifaceted.

The role of pharmaceutical companies, which have aggressively marketed hyperactivity drugs for half a century, must also be considered. Curtailing the ability of such companies to influence both the medical community and the general public through their advertising would be a sensible step to a more balanced approach to public health, as Rasmussen has argued with respect to other amphetamines.[119] Ritalin also conceals the fact that behaviours such as hyperactivity, impulsivity and inattentiveness may be positive in many situations outside the confines of a rigid classroom. Before drugs are employed to curtail a child's energy, initiative and creativity, perhaps it is incumbent upon us to consider changing his/her academic, social, physical and emotional environment. It may be more difficult to set up more active, child-centred classrooms, to offer children more physical exercise and better nutrition, to provide informal counselling and to ensure that children have a healthy home environment than it is to prescribe a pill, but it could be more effective and humane in the long run.

FIVE

Alternative Approaches

Biological explanations and pharmaceutical treatments for hyper-activity might have become predominant by the 1970s, but that did not mean that every parent – or physician – was satisfied with such approaches to the disorder. In 1978, an article in *Utah Holiday*, for example, told the story of a five-year-old girl whose hyperactivity was 'calmed . . . slightly' by a stimulant drug, but only at the expense of 'hallucinations, nightmares, insomnia, headaches, and less appetite'.[1] Another family described in the article had adopted three hyperactive children, one of whom was 'bent on pyromania'. Ritalin was prescribed for their children, but it 'would wear off in two hours and then the children would be even wilder'.[2] For these Utah parents, Ritalin was not the answer. Other parents had different reasons for questioning the conventional biological approach to hyperactivity. While some had read reports critical of hyperactivity medication and did not feel comfortable giving drugs to their child, others simply wanted to try some other options before resorting to stimulant medication.

Fortunately for these parents, as well as their sympathetic physi-cians, there were a number of alternative therapies from which to choose by the mid-1970s. Possible explanations for hyperactivity attributed its rising rates to everything from fluorescent lighting and food additives to television and lack of exercise in the great outdoors. One apparently serious letter writer to *American Psychologist* attributed some cases of hyperactivity to tight and itchy underwear, stating that a college student of his went from being a C to an A student once he began changing his underwear every day, rather than every two weeks.[3]

Even more alternative approaches to hyperactivity have emerged in the medical literature in the last couple of decades, reflecting both dissatisfaction with the conventional wisdom regarding the disorder and increasing interest in non-traditional medicine more generally. A review article by L. Eugene Arnold in 2001, for example, listed 24 alternative treatments for hyperactivity, including additive-free diets, herbal therapies, vitamin, amino acid and mineral supplementation, massage, meditation, acupuncture and electromyography (EMG) biofeedback.[4] While the efficacy of many of these therapies was based on a small number of clinical observations, other alternative approaches to hyperactivity had been studied in depth, some with promising results. But even in cases where a good deal of support was garnered through clinical and trial evidence, most physicians remained highly sceptical of such alternatives and ushered parents with hyperactive children firmly towards stimulant medication.

To a degree, the reluctance to consider alternative measures, especially untested ones, was understandable. For physicians in the 1970s who were intent on helping their hyperactive patients efficiently, stimulant therapy was simply seen as the best and most reliable approach to dealing with the disorder. When the countless advertisements for hyperactivity drugs in medical journals, inducements from pharmaceutical companies, positive results from clinical trials, and, most likely, a good number of success stories were taken into consideration by the average general practitioner, paediatrician or psychiatrist, it is not surprising that a prescription for Ritalin was their first port of call. Moreover, while the pharmaceutical treatment of hyperactivity fitted into a biomedical paradigm with which most physicians would feel comfortable, most alternatives were based on medical theories that took physicians out of their intellectual comfort zone. This is because unorthodox hypotheses about hyperactivity were typically rooted in ecological, nutritional or allergy theories that were regarded as controversial at best, and at worst, quackery. To abandon the mainstream approach for seemingly radical solutions promoted by those outside of the traditional sphere of mental health was to take a step too far for most psychiatrists, paediatricians and general practitioners.

Many frustrated parents, in addition to curious or empathetic physicians, however, thought otherwise and, when the context of the 1970s is considered, it is equally understandable that they might have done. During these years concern about ecology, the safety of the food supply and the dangers of pollution was widespread. Although research in the growing science of environmental toxicology helps to explain the connection, what really allied such fears with the notion that food, chemicals and other substances could trigger behavioural problems was a series of decades-old theories emanating from the field of allergy. Almost as soon as allergy was established in the early twentieth century, a subsection of the field became convinced that allergens, particularly those found in food, could cause mental illness.[5] Food allergists, therefore, worked with patients to identify the foods responsible for such problems and then prescribed elimination diets to prevent subsequent reactions. An article in 1922, for instance, described an eight-year-old boy who was 'extremely irritable, did not eat well, was cruel to his playmates, and was unable to apply himself at school', with the result that he had to repeat the first grade. After 'wheat, spinach, egg white, whole egg, pear, orange, pea, beef and figs' were eliminated from his diet, the boy's 'irritability was lessened; he was no longer cruel to his playmates; he was doing well in school'.[6]

Dozens of allergists reported similar cases, often describing such reactions as 'cerebral allergy' or 'neuroallergy'. A survey conducted by New York allergist T. Wood Clarke in 1950, entitled 'The Relation of Allergy to Character Problems in Children', indicated that out of the 171 allergists surveyed, 95 acknowledged 'that they had noticed personality changes due to allergy which corrected themselves when the allergic element was eliminated'.[7] Clarke described how the 40 anecdotes which accompanied his survey told of

> irritable, fretful, quarrelsome children, who could not get along with others, often had to be taken out of school as they upset the classes and were considered incorrigible, who, after the nature of their allergy was discovered and proper steps taken to correct it, became friendly and happy and took active and joyous part in the occupations of their mates.[8]

Others, including Kansas City allergist Frederic Speer, also claimed that behavioural problems resembling hyperactivity were a form of allergic reaction. Speer's 'allergic tension fatigue syndrome' was often a reaction to foods such as chocolate, milk and corn, as well as synthetic food dyes, moulds and pollens.[9]

Given the similarity of such descriptions to those of hyperactive children a decade later, it is striking that early hyperactivity researchers made scant reference to the experiences of food allergists, preferring to link their observations to those of researchers studying post-encephalitic disorder and organic brain damage. But while theories of 'cerebral allergy' or 'allergic tension fatigue syndrome' might have impressed many allergists, they were nonetheless very controversial and became increasingly so during the 1950s and 1960s as the field of allergy, much like psychiatry, sought to become more scientifically respectable.[10] By the 1960s a number of these unorthodox allergists, led by Theron G. Randolph (1906–1995), had split from mainstream allergy to form the new discipline of clinical ecology, which was concerned chiefly with the chronic health problems believed to be caused by environmental and nutritional factors. Randolph, who had previously described how food allergies could trigger behavioural problems in children, was convinced that 'foods, insecticide residues on food, fumes from gas ranges and many other non-personal environmental physical exposures are common demonstrable causes of mental and behavioural disturbances'.[11] Although Randolph's views were divisive and brought him into conflict with the American Academy of Allergy, his then-employer, Northwestern University, and most of his fellow allergists, his empirical, individualized approach also won him many admirers, particularly among his patients, whose chronic ailments had often been dismissed as being psychosomatic in nature.

The divisive nature of food allergy and clinical ecology meant that nutritional and environmental theories of hyperactivity were often lambasted, particularly after the psychiatric debates about the nature of hyperactivity had been won by biological psychiatrists. There were few exceptions to this. Theories linking lead exposure to hyperactivity, for example, gained a good deal of traction during the early 1970s, partly due to the broader demonization of such substances during this period, but also because some clinicians noted that hyperactive children were more likely to have accidentally come into contact with poisons early in life.[12] As one neurologist described:

> I originally got interested in lead because of children who had lead poisoning and had been sent home from the hospital cured, who then turned up in my neurological clinic because they were misbehaving in one way or another or not learning in school . . . They all had evidence of lead poisoning [and] when they reached six or seven, they showed evidence of neurologic injury.[13]

Although the level of lead required to call such disturbances was difficult to determine, many researchers believed that quite low levels would be sufficient, possibly so low that the more common clinical symptoms of lead poisoning would be absent.[14] Other researchers developed experiments using animal models which provided additional evidence for the association.[15] For psychiatrist Oliver J. David, the link between lead and hyperactivity was strong enough for him to argue that inquiries about lead levels 'should be routine investigations in cases of hyperactivity', adding that the social and public health implications of such findings were 'staggering'.[16]

Not all physicians were quite as impressed. A letter writer to the Lancet, for example, suggested that the link could be one of correlation rather than causation. In other words, 'the raised lead levels may be a consequence of the child's hyperactivity rather than the cause of the hyperactivity'.[17] Different animal experiments were also conducted, finding little evidence in favour of the hypothesis.[18] The debate continued in subsequent decades, although new American legislation restricting lead-based paints (1978) and in leaded petrol (beginning in 1975) somewhat muted its urgency. Recent research, however, has renewed interest in the association, including a degree of media attention.[19] Still, the hypothesis never became as contentious or inflammatory as those linking hyperactivity with food allergy. This is due in part to the fact that lead has long been

associated with toxic effects, including those affecting the neurological system. Similarly, biofeedback, vitamin and fish oil treatment of hyperactivity have also generated a small degree of serious
medical interest, possibly because they have been seen as being
beneficial in other conditions.[20]

The same cannot be said for the link between food additives and
hyperactivity. Among all of the alternative explanations for hyperactivity, the most infamous, controversial, yet enduring was that of
San Francisco allergist Benjamin F. Feingold (1899–1982), who
began treating hyperactive children in the early 1970s with an
elimination diet free of synthetic colours and flavours. Although
Feingold's theory and the so-called Feingold diet was compelling
to the media and the general public, due to contemporary concerns
about food additives and dissatisfaction with conventional
approaches to hyperactivity, the medical community was unim-
pressed and soon began designing trials to test his hypothesis. The
prevailing opinion emerging out of the trials was that the Feingold
diet was not an effective treatment for hyperactivity.

The history of the Feingold diet is a strange chapter in the
broader history of hyperactivity, the ending of which has not yet
been written. It is as much about the history of food, allergy,
environmentalism and the nature of scientific knowledge as it is
about psychiatry and hyperactivity, and has been discussed in detail
elsewhere.[21] When juxtaposed against other developments in how
hyperactivity has been understood and experienced, however, the
story of the Feingold diet demonstrates how ideology and economic
expediency have often trumped clinical and scientific evidence in
the debates about which factors contribute to hyperactive behaviour.
Specifically, when the trials designed to test the Feingold diet are
examined in detail, it is difficult to see how such firm conclusions
were made based on the evidence the trials provided. Many of the
trials were beset by methodological problems, were often funded
by those with vested interests and were questionably interpreted by
both Feingold's supporters and detractors. Moreover, thousands of
parents found the Feingold diet to be effective in minimizing the
hyperactivity of their children, yet their experiences and observations were ignored. In many ways, the manner in which Feingold's

hypothesis was tested, judged and ultimately rejected by most physicians highlights the medical community's unwillingness to consider seriously any unorthodox theories of hyperactivity, particularly after the genetic, neurological explanations for, and stimulant treatment of, the disorder were firmly established during the early 1970s.

Why Your Child Is Hyperactive

Although it is almost certain that Feingold had been familiar with the link between food allergy and childhood behavioural problems long before he devised his famous diet, he claimed to have first made the connection in 1965, after treating a middle-aged woman for hives.[22] Feingold had recently seen cases where artificial food additives had been responsible for such symptoms and, after determining that the woman was not allergic to any other allergens which typically caused hives, prescribed a diet free of such substances. Within a few days the hives had disappeared. A week later Feingold, who was chief of allergy at the Kaiser Permanente Health Center, received a call from his opposite number in the psychiatry department. After discovering what Feingold had prescribed, the psychiatrist revealed that the woman had also been a patient of his, and had been presenting aggressive and hostile behaviour for years. Since starting the elimination diet, these behaviours had disappeared, along with the hives.

In the years that followed, Feingold noted other patients whose 'personality disturbances' were alleviated when food additives were removed from their diet.[23] Having conducted research into the allergenicity of low-molecular-weight chemicals during the 1950s, Feingold began to suspect that a similarly low-weight group of chemicals, called salicylates, might be responsible for such reactions. Such salicylates were not only found in synthetic colours and flavours, but also occurred naturally in fruits and vegetables, such as tomatoes, grapes and apples. He also began to read about the growing epidemic of hyperactivity that was sweeping North America. Feingold reported being 'alarmed' and 'shocked' by the numbers of children diagnosed with hyperactivity, as well as the 'frightening but often necessary drug management'.[24] Noting that the proliferation of food additives was a post-war phenomenon, just like the hyperactivity epidemic, Feingold began to wonder if the two were connected. Believing that his additive-free diet might help hyperactive children, he began prescribing it regularly in the early 1970s and soon he was convinced that it worked.

It did not take long for Feingold's hypothesis to attract attention. By 1972 he was discussing his theory on San Francisco television and in the spring of 1973 he was invited by the American Medical Association (AMA) to present his theory not only to their members, but also at a press conference they organized. The media took hold of the story and soon stories about the Feingold diet were being published regularly in major newspapers and magazines.[25] One story, published in the *Washington Post* by the journalist who broke the thalidomide scandal, Morton Mintz, was reprinted verbatim in the *Congressional Record*, and political attention subsequently followed.[26] Parents dissatisfied with pharmaceutical treatments for hyperactivity and desperate for alternatives were also captivated by Feingold's idea, and Feingold Associations, providing support, advice and information to Feingold families, sprang up across the US and elsewhere.

Although Feingold initially received encouragement from the AMA, who invited him to speak again in 1974, support from them and the broader medical community soon waned. Feingold had previously published dozens of articles in leading medical journals on topics including bronchial allergy, flea-bite allergy and psychosomatic aspects of allergy, and had recently published a highly acclaimed textbook on clinical allergy.[27] But when he sent articles to the *Journal of the American Medical Association* (JAMA), the *British Medical Journal* (BMJ) and the *Western Journal of Medicine*, his submissions were rejected.[28] Given his reputation as a leading California allergist, his position within Kaiser Permanente, his nearly 50 years of clinical experience, his previous publication record and his admittedly high opinion of himself, Feingold was not only dejected, but also shocked by this negative response. Feingold dealt with this rebuff from the medical community by turning attention to the public and, specifically, parents. When the publishing giant

Random House offered to publish his ideas in a popular book, Feingold decided to seize the opportunity.

The resulting *Why Your Child Is Hyperactive* (1974) and *The Feingold Cookbook for Hyperactive Children* (1979) were best-sellers, the latter reaching fourth place on the *New York Times* list of non-fiction trade paperbacks. Feingold's publishing successes and his emerging status as a television and radio celebrity did little to endear him to the medical community. What many hyperactivity experts found particularly irksome was that Feingold had failed to conduct randomly controlled trials to test his hypothesis, relying instead on his clinical observations. Feingold's reasons for eschewing such tests were threefold. First, Feingold was in his seventies and was in failing health, having survived cancer and heart disease, and feared that he would not live long enough to see the results of such trials. Second, Feingold had experienced frustrations designing similar trials to test a flea-bite allergy extract that would be suitable for clinical desensitization during the 1950s and 1960s. Although his research had made important theoretical contributions to immunology, Feingold found the difficulty in designing a trial that would indubitably prove the efficacy of the extract exasperating. Finally, the more Feingold prescribed the diet and heard success stories from parents, the more he was determined that such tests were unnecessary. As he would state on a radio broadcast: 'I don't have time for sacred cows of science, the double-blind placebo controlled trials.'[29]

Unsurprisingly, many physicians were not satisfied with such excuses. John S. Werry, a New Zealand child psychiatrist who had also worked in Montreal, expressed his resentment bluntly in criticizing Feingold's decision to publicize his theory before conducting controlled trials:

I personally feel there is no greater breach of medical ethics than that of foisting a potentially worthless or dangerous treatment on to a credulous public. Theirs may be the right to believe in magic and panaceas but ours as a profession is to act responsibly, cautiously and scientifically, though not prejudicially. Why should all of my u.s. colleagues in paediatric psychopharmacology research, no more than a handful, have to drop their work to show a clamouring public that Feingold's hypothesis is or is not correct and is or is not safe? Surely the obligation is his before he announces it to the public?[30]

Most physicians agreed with such sentiments and soon a series of controlled trials were designed to test Feingold's hypothesis. Among those involved in the trials was a food, chemical and pharmaceutical lobby group called the Nutrition Foundation, which had been created in 1941 and was often 'used to marshal scientific opinions to correct "superficial and faddish ideas" questioning any of the 704 chemicals that by 1958 were commonly used in foods'.[31] Not only did the Nutrition Foundation, whose previous targets had included Rachel Carson and Silent Spring (1962), fund and supply many trials, they also organized a task force, the National Advisory Committee on Hyperkinesis and Food Additives (NACHFA), to review the trials and assess their findings.[32]

By the time of Feingold's death in 1982, most of the medical community, NACHFA and the American Council on Science and Health (ACSH), a non-profit consumer education group with ties to the food industry, all agreed that the trials provided little evidence in support of Feingold's hypothesis.[33] Any effects, it was argued, were likely due to placebo effect; changing routines in the household, in addition to the added attention given to the hyperactive child and the benign, grandfatherly influence of Feingold himself, were thought to be more responsible than a change in diet. Given that most physicians believed that hyperactivity was fundamentally neurological deficit, this focus on changes within the family might seem rather odd, but it does underline how Feingold's detractors were willing to attack him on numerous fronts. Other reasons for dismissing the diet were also offered, with much attention paid to the practicality of the diet. The additional shopping, label reading and meal preparation were thought to place undue strain on families who were already struggling with the burden of a hyperactive child. Some researchers also claimed that children would not receive enough vitamin C while on the Feingold diet, since many fruits were eliminated during the early stages of the diet, only to be reintroduced when it was determined that they were not causing any reactions.[34] Finally, the willingness of impulsive, distractible children to stick to the diet was also questioned; how would they cope with Halloween and birthday parties? Even if the Feingold diet was efficacious, NACHFA, ACSH and the Nutrition Foundation argued that it was impossible to employ.

Without the charismatic San Francisco allergist leading the way, the impetus behind his idea was lost. Feingold, who for most of his career had been an orthodox allergist and, as such, was 'leery of "cure" by diet', did not endear himself to food allergists and clinical ecologists, such as Randolph, who could have been natural allies, and so few, apart from the parent-led Feingold Association of the United States (FAUS), carried on his mission after his death.[35] In addition, the media of the 1980s had moved on to a certain extent from the food fears of the late 1960s and 1970s. Health food during the 1980s became more about products that were low in fat, carbohydrates and sugar, rather than those which were free of chemicals. Although many of the small number of trials conducted after 1982 were better designed and most provided support for Feingold's hypothesis, they tended to receive little media coverage. The Feingold diet moved from exciting possibility to food fad in the medical, media and popular imagination and, for most physicians, and most families with hyperactive children, it ceased to be a viable treatment option for hyperactive children.

Troublesome Trials

But it was not clear whether bodies such as the Nutrition Foundation, as well as physicians, the media and the general public had reached the correct decision about Feingold's hypothesis. One hint of this was the findings of a National Institutes for Health (NIH) Consensus Development Conference in 1982, whose participants included both an ailing Feingold and his critics. Although the panel stated that 'defined diets should not be universally used in the treatment of childhood hyperactivity at this time', it also indicated that 'initiation of a trial of dietary treatment or continuation of a diet in patients whose families and physicians perceive benefits, may be warranted' in some cases.[36] The panel also stressed the need for more trials, including both epidemiological and animal studies, in order to resolve the issue definitively. According to the NIH, the jury was still out on the matter.

When the tests of the Feingold diet are examined carefully, it is difficult not to come to this conclusion. A quick look at the literature reveals that, while there were negative results, there were also plenty of positive results and other trials which were inconclusive. A longer look demonstrates that few of the trials were without design flaws, leading to questions about why researchers made bold conclusions based on inconclusive data. The many methodological problems included ensuring the trials would be blind and controlled, determining what substances would be tested, measuring the changes in child behaviour and maintaining the compliance of the subjects. The Feingold diet might have been a 'difficult and exacting regimen' for families, but it was even harder to test.[37]

The first task of researchers testing the Feingold diet was to eliminate any possibility of the placebo effect influencing their findings. As explained above, many of Feingold's critics believed that the benefits of the Feingold diet were not due to the diet itself, but instead caused by placebo. As such, the trials had to be double blind; neither the participants nor the researchers should know which children were on the additive-free diet and which were on the control diet. In addition, all aspects of the participants' lives that might affect their behaviour were also controlled as much as possible. Guaranteeing this, however, was not particularly easy.

The first problem was determining what aspects of the Feingold diet should be tested. Although the diet included a wide range of colours, flavours, preservatives and fruits and vegetables, even Feingold acknowledged that it would be easier to focus on the synthetic food dyes. While this meant that not all aspects of his diet would be tested, leaving the potential for outliers (children who reacted especially to preservatives or flavours, for example) to be overlooked, it was hoped that the tests might contribute to more rigorously controlled trials. But even testing food colours alone proved to be complicated. The first issue was the amount of dye to be tested. As part of determining the parameters for the trials that it supported, NACHFA designed a test cookie, which it supplied to researchers. The amount of dye in these cookies was based upon a calculation of the average daily per capita consumption of the nine most common food dyes in the United States during the years 1973 and 1974. The amount of each dye used was proportional to their overall consumption, meaning that some dyes, such as indigotine (Blue Number 2) only made up 1.7 per cent of the total amount of dyes in the cookie. One of the problems with this rather blunt measurement, as NACHFA admitted, was that children were not only smaller than adults, but also consumed more food additives on average in the form of candy, soft drinks and processed snacks.[38] Or as psychologist and autism researcher Bernard Rimland (1926–2008) exclaimed:

> The dosage levels were ridiculously small. Even if one were to accept the wholly unwarranted conclusion that seven to 10 food colorings were the overwhelming important factor in the Feingold diet, one would still have to reject the bulk of the studies, since the researchers used almost trivially small doses of colorings.[39]

Rimland's charges notwithstanding, it is more accurate to say that dosage levels varied wildly across studies; while one study's materials only contained 1.2 mg of dye, another study subjected participants to 150 mg. Strangely, both of these studies yielded positive results.[40] NACHFA originally expected children in the studies it supported to eat two of its test cookies, containing 26 mg in total. The committee realized, however, that this might be too little and subsequently designed 'a soda pop drink' that contained 36 mg.[41] But this amount was also below the FDA average of 57.5 mg, and far below FDA estimates of what children at the high end of the spectrum might consume, namely, as much 121 mg for children in the ninetieth percentile and rising up to a maximum of 315 mg per day.[42] When this was combined with the fact that dyes such as indigotine represented a tiny amount of the dyes in the cookies, it resulted in the possibility that some trial participants were being exposed to infinitesimal amounts of the dye to which they might be particularly reactive. Nevertheless, when criticized over the amount of dye in their materials NACHFA responded that there was 'a technical limitation to the amount of food coloring that can be incorporated into a food without coloring the mouth and fingers . . . and thus preventing the disguise of the placebo challenge'.[43] Given the availability of numerous natural food dyes, including saffron (yellow), betanin (red/purple), butterfly pea (blue) and pandan (green), and the willingness of other researchers to overcome such difficulties, however, such protestations fell flat in the eyes of Feingold's supporters.

Investigators also differed about how the behaviour of children in the trials should be assessed. This is not particularly surprising given the subjective nature of hyperactivity. Discrepancies existed regarding how to identify all the different components of hyper-active behaviour, including distractibility, impulsivity, defiance and aggression. Although Conners's parent and teacher questionnaires, designed during the 1960s by psychologist C. Keith Conners, were used in many trials, observers could differ with respect to what was pathological, disordered behaviour and what constituted energetic play. As an anonymous editorial for the Lancet observed, Feingold's 'hypothesis would be difficult to test even if the state of hyperactivity in children were a precise and readily recognisable entity. It is not.'[44]

In one influential trial, conducted by University of Wisconsin psychologist J. Preston Harley, for example, the results of an entire sample set was dismissed because of the difficulty in distinguish-ing hyperactive behaviour. Harley's study, which was funded by the Nutrition Foundation, tested the Feingold diet on two groups of children, one consisting of 36 boys aged between six and twelve years old and another consisting of ten preschool-aged boys. Although the Nutrition Foundation's support (estimated at $120 per week per family) meant that his trial was well designed and con-ducted, Harley decided to reject the preschool sample, despite the fact that: 'All ten mothers and four of the seven fathers of the pre-school sample rated their children's behavior as improved on the experimental diet.'[45] Harley's rationale for rejecting the preschool sample was that these trials were based on parental, rather than parental and teacher, rating scales, and that it was more difficult to gauge hyperactivity in preschoolers. This decision was particularly questionable, given the observations of Feingold and other researchers that younger children responded especially well to additive-free diets, and left some researchers wondering if Harley had been unduly influenced by his funders.[46] Or as Conners contended:

> they cannot have it both ways. If their study did indeed rigorously achieve a complete disguise of the dietary manipulations, then the parent ratings, regardless of their 'subjectivity' have to be explained. The probability of obtaining such findings by chance alone is miniscule.[47]

Conners's critique of Harley's interpretation of the parental findings is interesting, partly because of his role in designing assessment tools for hyperactivity, but also because his own opinion about the Feingold diet vacillated considerably. The psychologist's struggle to arrive at a firm decision about Feingold's hypothesis suggests how challenging it was to test, but also raises the question of why other researchers were so assured about their own findings.

The final methodological problem involved the children who participated in the trials and their ability and willingness to persevere through trials that could take weeks to complete. According to the authors of one trial set in a summer camp for children with learning disabilities:

> One result was unmistakable: the children were not happy with the Feingold diet. The teachers had the feeling that there would have been a rebellion had it lasted longer than a week. They particularly disliked the colourlessness of the food, and missed the mustard and ketchup. . . . The strict Feingold diet appears to be distasteful to the typical American child.[48]

Ironically, the authors conducted their trial at a summer camp in order to reduce infractions, but this did not prevent their study from being marred by a long list of methodological problems, including the fact that many of the children involved were not actually hyperactive, the manner in which their behaviour was observed and the controls in place. Perseverance was also an issue, despite the confined environment, with three participants being sent home for behavioural problems during the week when the additives were reintroduced to their diet. Although the authors claimed the diet was 'distasteful' to children and suspected a 'rebellion' was likely if it was continued, the conclusion of the camp director and teachers was that the children had behaved better during the week it was introduced.

Many other studies struggled to ensure that its participants, and their parents, complied with the rigorous conditions of double-blind controlled trials. Compliance could be undermined by both infractions, when children managed to eat additive-laden food surreptitiously, and by parents removing their children from the study during the challenge phase, when additives were reintro-duced. Compliance was also a matter of opinion. While Harley believed that the 1.33 infractions per week he reported would not affect his overall findings, Feingold argued that a single infraction could disrupt a child's behaviour for up to six days, meaning that Harley's results had in fact been compromised.[49] In another case, a participant struggled to consume daily the six test cookies demanded of her by the researchers.[50] Disturbed by the reactions they perceived in their children after eating so many cookies, two sets of parents removed their children from this study, but only one of the children was actually eating cookies with synthetic food colours; the other had been consuming placebo cookies. Although other factors, including the sugar present in six cookies, might have also explained some of the behavioural problems witnessed by these parents, many others removed their children from the trials, believ-ing that the additives were harming their children, when in fact they were consuming the placebo.[51] Such removals hampered the statis-tical significance of trials, particularly when they included a small number of participants.

While it was inherently difficult to test the Feingold diet, the willingness of researchers to design and conduct methodologically sound trials is less apparent. Some observers argued that poorly designed trials were carried out by people who thought they already knew the answers to the questions they were asking. Others, such as

Canadian researchers J. Ivan Williams and Douglas M. Cram, commented that 'there has been interest in testing [the Feingold hypothesis] if only to disprove it', suggesting that ensuring a sound methodological approach might not have been overly important to some researchers.[52] The existence of well-designed trials, in addition, also indicates that testing the Feingold diet in a sophisticated, meticulous manner was possible. One trial, conducted by Bonnie Kaplan at the University of Calgary, for example, overcame many of the methodological challenges by integrating a 'dietary replacement design'.[53] This involved comparing the behavioural effects of an additive-laden diet with one free of such substances, instead of testing only a small number of synthetic colours. Such an approach was complicated and expensive, but Kaplan, unlike most of those involved in the trials, saw it as an exciting challenge, rather than an opportunity to praise or criticize Feingold's idea. Flabbergasted by the poor quality of the previous trials and claiming to have no preconceived notions about what the results would be, Kaplan believed that she could do a better job, and according to many observers, did just that.

'Arbitrary Negative Conclusions'?

What is most interesting about Kaplan's study is not necessarily her findings, which provided modest support for the Feingold diet, but her interpretation of her results and their broader implications. She described how

> On the one hand, a much larger percentage of children responded to dietary intervention than was found in previous studies. On the other hand, only half of the children who completed the study exhibited behavioral improvement, and it is safe to say that not a single parent believed that participation in this study had transformed their child into an easy to manage person.[54]

Kaplan's balanced summary differed from both Feingold's supporters and detractors, who often saw the diet in starker, more definitive, terms. This was certainly the case with the reviews of the research into the Feingold diet. Whether these were statistical meta-analyses or more informal assessments, the reviewers appeared to make their judgements by picking and choosing studies that supported their view. While psychiatrist Jeffrey Mattes contended that the diet was a 'fad', and that concerns about the effect additives had on behaviour were 'unwarranted', others, such as Bernard Rimland, accused researchers of making 'arbitrary negative conclusions'.[55] So, which reviewers were correct?

The answer, as with most related to the history of hyperactivity, is difficult to judge. But it is strange how few investigators recognized this. What is striking about the debates concerning the Feingold diet is how the majority of researchers and observers seemed determined to view the Feingold diet as an either/or proposition. Measured opinions, such as those offered by Kaplan, or changing views, exemplified by Conners's difficulty in determining whether the diet was effective or not, were a rarity, rather than the norm. Instead, most of those involved in the debates expressed their views unequivocally. Hyperactivity was either caused by food additives or it was not. An additive-free diet was either a godsend or it was a pernicious imposition on families. There was seemingly little room for the possibility that food additives might trigger hyperactive behaviour in a small number of the children so-diagnosed or that such behaviour might be exacerbated to varying degrees by synthetic colours, additives and preservatives.

Why was this the case? Although the role of the Nutrition Foundation and other interested parties might be implicated, it is more likely that the medical ideologies held by those involved were the critical factors. If one had spent years researching the genetic and neurological aspects of hyperactivity and believed that it was best treated with stimulants, possibly applying such theories in one's clinical practice, Feingold's theory might be thought to contain an ominous undercurrent. The words of John S. Werry, for example, betrayed a palpable fear that the Feingold diet would threaten the newly established biological paradigm in psychiatry:

> the most chilling aspect of Feingold's work lies in the enthusiasm with which it has been embraced by the anti-

medication, anti-psychiatry section of the American public
and used as a cudgel to try to close down paediatric psychopharmacological research.[56]

Feingold, according to Werry, was nothing more than a 'medical
pied piper', leading children, their parents and even some physicians away from the true causes and treatments of hyperactivity.[57]

In contrast, those who had long believed in the link between
food additives and behaviour, such as the food allergist William G.
Crook (1917–2002), believed that while 'many physicians remain
sceptical or even hostile' to Feingold's idea: 'I know, beyond any
shadow of a doubt, based on what my patients tell me, that many,
and perhaps most, hyperactive children can be helped by changing
their diets.'[58] As with many other aspects of the history of hyperactivity, what was lost in the debates about the Feingold diet was any
sense that the disorder could be caused or worsened by multiple
factors. Children's behaviour is seen only from one, ideologically
entrenched, perspective, rather than being perceived as complex,
mercurial and affected by numerous changes in the social, familial
and, indeed, physical environment.

Ironically, Feingold himself acknowledged that hyperactivity
and behavioural problems generally had familial and, particularly,
social dimensions. For him it was the case that

> Without question, socioeconomic pressures influence in-
> stinctive behaviour, and such behaviour becomes imprinted
> on the patterns of the individual. It is rather easily identifi-
> able and does not need a psychologist's explanation.
> Deprived infanthood and adolescence can add up to [sic]
> troubled adult.[59]

But:

> these factors do not now provide the complete answer to the
> sharp upward curve of aggression and violence of the past
> twenty-five years. The ghetto can no longer claim sole
> ownership. The attack by fist, knife and gun has spread to

the stamping grounds of the middle class and into wealthy suburbia; the snarl of frustration and rage spills out universally and from unlikely mouths.[60]

Although Feingold believed passionately in the effectiveness of his diet, he was also convinced that hyperactivity was a 'multifactorial reaction between the genetic profile and an environmental activator'. In other words, problematic behaviour was the admixture of numerous circumstances, many of which were difficult to control or predict. While food additives could be the primary trigger, an overcrowded classroom could also be a contributory factor.[61] It is possible that, had more American psychiatrists agreed that hyperactivity was a multidimensional phenomenon, the Feingold diet would have been much less controversial and, instead, viewed as yet another facet of what was a complicated and recalcitrant disorder.

Lost in and among the furore over the trials and competing ideologies were the experiences of families who had actually tried the diet.[62] It was estimated that, by 1983, 200,000 families had tried the diet and 20,000 families were members of regional Feingold Associations, which would eventually conglomerate into FAUS.[63] Many parents had turned to the diet as an act of desperation, when they found that conventional explanations and treatments for hyperactivity did not help their child. Although some families were unable to cope with the rigours of the diet, reading labels carefully, preparing additive-free meals and controlling what their child ate at home, school, the corner store and at their friends' houses, thousands found it to be effective and, in large part, kept the Feingold's diet alive long after he had died. In many cases, the children who were first put on the Feingold diet during the 1970s now employ an additive-free diet in their own homes, meaning that some families have employed it for nearly 40 years. While many parents admitted that the Feingold diet was often part of a larger strategy to combat their child's hyperactivity – some children were sent to more accommodating schools or were home-schooled, for example – all were convinced that eliminating food additives had a fundamental impact on their child's behaviour. Despite the inherent problems in testing the Feingold diet in controlled trials and the countless methodological issues that emerged, however, the experiences of Feingold families played little role in shaping the opinions of medical professionals.

In 2004, 30 years after the publication of *Why Your Child Is Hyperactive*, interest in the Feingold diet emerged once again. Responding to public pressure, the British Food Standards Agency (FSA) solicited proposals to test the relationship between food additives and children's behaviour. A group led by University of Southampton psychologist Jim Stevenson was given funding and designed a trial testing 277 children from the Isle of Wight. Parental rating scales indicated that 'significant changes in children's hyperactive behaviour could be produced by the removal of artificial colourings and sodium benzoate from their diet' and the researchers concluded that 'benefit would accrue for all children if artificial food colours and benzoate preservatives were removed from their diet'.[64]

The research team's report in the *Archives of Disease in Childhood* only received limited publicity, but a second trial, published in the prestigious *Lancet*, put the Feingold diet on the front pages of newspapers once again. Again, their findings provided 'strong support for the case that food additives exacerbate hyperactive behaviours . . . in children at least up to middle childhood' and showed that such increases were 'not just seen in children with extreme hyperactivity (that is, ADHD) but also can be seen in the general population and across the range of severities of hyperactivity'.[65] The authors' comments, that the 'implications of these results for the regulation of food additive use could be substantial', proved to be prophetic, as the FSA and the European Food Safety Authority (EFSA) both revised their guidelines for the consumption of certain food colours.[66] Included in the changes to EFSA policy was that foods or drinks which contained six of the major synthetic colours had to include a label stating that they 'may have an adverse effect on activity and attention in children'.[67]

American physicians, policy makers and, indeed, the American media were slower to respond to the new findings. One exception was found in a summary of the *Lancet* article made by the American Academy of Pediatrics, which had long criticized Feingold's hypothesis. In the accompanying editorial, paediatrician Alison Schonwald praised the trial and its implications for clinical paediatric practice and concluded that

> the overall findings of the study are clear and require that even we skeptics, who have long doubted parental claims of the effects of various foods on the behavior of their children, admit we might have been wrong.[68]

Although it might be thought that such an admission would have prompted regulatory action in the United States which mirrored what had been put in place in Europe, this was not to be. The FDA did organize a panel to discuss the matter in March 2011, but, on the basis of a narrow 8-to-6 vote, decided not to mandate the labelling of foods containing food colours. The lack of enough rigorous studies and data was cited as the primary reason for delaying any action on food dyes, and the panel called for more research to be done.[69] In other words, despite dozens of trials and the experiences of thousands of families, the medical community remained undecided about whether or not there was a link between hyperactivity and food additives.

The protracted debates about the Feingold diet are instructive in many ways. They demonstrate how difficult it is to prove definitively the validity of novel medical theories, particularly when they involve food and behaviour, and when they contradict already established ideas. They also highlight the gap which can exist between clinical and patient experience, which fuelled Feingold's efforts and those of FAUS after he died, and the kind of knowledge made authoritative by randomly controlled double-blind trials. To a large degree, they show how interest in new medical hypotheses is often driven by historical and cultural trends. British interest in the Feingold diet in the late 1990s and 2000s was driven, for example, by food supply disasters, such as BSE and foot-and-mouth disease, and deteriorating confidence in mainstream medicine, exemplified by the MMR and autism debate. But as an episode within the history of hyperactivity, the history of the Feingold diet illuminates how limited and inflexible understandings of the disorder could be.

Rather than embracing the possibility that children's behaviour could be affected by the foods they consumed, a phenomenon acknowledged by food allergists for decades, hyperactivity experts sought to undermine and disprove Feingold's theory. It remains to be seen whether the millions of children prescribed Ritalin during the second half of the twentieth century should have been prescribed an additive-free diet instead.

SIX

Hyperactive Around the World

In 2007, the first World Congress on ADHD, organized by the equally impressive-sounding ADHD World Federation, was held in Würtzburg, Germany. Boasting presentations from 'all continents', the topics for discussion ranged from using fruit flies to model cognitive disorders to using 'Cartoons about ADHD for Children as a Method of Psychoeducation'. Although the most represented countries, according to the presentations given, unsurprisingly included the US and Germany, given the location of the conference, other countries listed in the top ten included Malaysia, Poland and Brazil. The Scientific Program Committee for the conference was similarly international, featuring members from China, Japan, Nigeria, Egypt, Romania and Turkey.

Despite representing such a wide range of countries, the Federation's conceptualization of ADHD was rather narrow. Specifically:

> ADHD is a highly heritable childhood-onset psychiatric condition which is characterized by age-inappropriate levels of the core symptoms inattention, hyperactivity and impulsivity. . . . Recent scientific studies in ADHD reveal biological underpinnings such as multiple genetic factors, ADHD-related differences in brain structure and function, as well as changes in neurotransmitter components within the basal ganglia thalamocortical neurocircuitries.[1]

Reflecting both this biological approach to the disorder, and the meeting's international flavour, the sponsors for the initial and subsequent congresses consisted primarily of pharmaceutical companies specializing in hyperactivity drugs, including New Jersey's Janssen Pharmaceuticals (Concerta), Belgium's UCB (Metadate), Germany's Medice (Medikinet), the UK's Shire (Adderall) and Switzerland's Novartis (Ritalin). Other sponsors included Qbtech, the Swedish manufacturer of Qbtest, a diagnostic test for hyperactivity, and Reha Klinik Neuharlingersiel, a German rehabilitation clinic for children with hyperactivity. Hyperactivity, it appears, has not only gone global, it is also globally profitable.

By the 2000s, epidemiological studies were also indicating that hyperactivity was a disorder that afflicted children – and adults – worldwide. In the same year as the first World Congress on ADHD, a Brazilian team of researchers calculated the global prevalence of hyperactivity. Attempting to explain why rates of hyperactivity varied so much from region to region, they pored through medical and psychological databases, examining epidemiological studies which discussed the disorder between the years 1978 and 2005. Calculating the figures, the team determined that hyperactivity occurred in 5.29 per cent of the world's childhood population. More importantly, they contended that variability in rates of hyperactivity were due to methodological differences between the studies rather than differences in the actual distribution of the disorder in different countries. In other words, hyperactive children were evenly distributed throughout the world; no one country had a monopoly over the disorder, as explained in an article by the Brazilian team in the *American Journal of Psychiatry*.[2] According to a commentary which accompanied the article, such findings gave weight to the status of the disorder's 'identity as a bona fide mental disorder ... as opposed to a social construction', and weakened assertions that hyperactivity was a 'fraud propagated by the profit-dependent pharmaceutical industry and a high-status profession (psychiatry) looking for new roles'.[3] This was despite the fact that the study itself was funded in part by pharmaceutical company Eli Lilly, for whom one of the authors, Silva de Lima, works as medical director. Two of the other authors were on the board of Eli Lilly and had ties to many other pharmaceutical companies, receiving funding from them and serving on their speakers' bureaus.[4] Nevertheless, a similar article (funded in part by Johnson and Johnson, another pharmaceutical company) contended that the worldwide prevalence of hyperactivity also undermined the notion that the disorder was 'largely an American disorder' rooted in 'social and cultural factors that are most common in American society'.[5]

The funding of such articles by pharmaceutical companies notwithstanding, these findings may be seen to jeopardize the argument that it is important to understand the origins and cultural aspects of hyperactivity in order to deal with the challenges it poses more effectively. The history of hyperactivity described here thus far has largely been an American story, featuring American physicians, parents and educators, with changes in American society playing a major role. This focus on the American context, however, is not accidental. When one considers how and why hyperactivity first emerged, examining the early years of the disorder, the story is clearly rooted in the US. There are simply very few discussions of hyperactive children in the non-American medical literature and, perhaps more importantly, the disorder is of little cultural significance outside of the US. The kind of stories about hyperactivity that emerge during the 1960s in Time, Life and the Washington Post are not replicated in the media to the same extent in other countries until later decades. Moreover, hyperactivity remained a largely North American concept for over twenty years following the diagnosis of the first hyperactive children in the late 1950s. This period, 1957–77, was not included in the Brazilian team's study, and no mention is made of why this was the case.[6] If it had been included it would have been dominated indubitably by North American studies. The researchers also failed to reveal the chronological distribution of the studies they did examine, leading to questions about when studies about hyperactivity did pop up in the international medical literature. How many non-American articles did they find during the first decade they examined, 1978–88? What about 1988–98? It is helpful to review epidemiological studies and use them to gauge the prevalence of particular disorders, but it is essential to determine when, where and why such diagnoses became worthy of discussion. As argued in chapter Two, a certain percentage of American children have always been overactive, impulsive and distractible, but it took until the late 1950s and the crisis in American education caused by *Sputnik* for such behaviour to be deemed worthy of a medical diagnosis, namely, hyperkinetic impulse disorder. Even if hyperactive behaviour was evenly distributed throughout the world's childhood population at a rate of 5.29 per cent, a prospect that will delight 'profit-dependent' pharmaceutical companies, this does not address why this was the case. Hyperactivity experts might posit that psychiatrists in Europe and Asia are only now becoming aware of the disorder's existence, but, given that hyperactivity is only thought to be pathological in certain situations, this rather arrogant explanation is not all that illuminating.

How did hyperactivity spread from being a largely American disorder to a condition that is diagnosed throughout the world? As with the history of hyperactivity in the US, there are multiple reasons for its dissemination, many of which are specific to particular countries. Although it is unfeasible to analyse how every country has discovered hyperactivity, the development of the disorder in two countries, Canada and the UK, will be explored, demonstrating how the international emergence of hyperactivity has resulted from an admixture of local factors and global trends even in countries with close connections to the US. The adoption of the American biomedical model of hyperactivity, therefore, has been tempered to a large degree by national circumstances and traditions. This should not be particularly surprising. Approaches to psychiatry and to childhood behavioural problems have often been shaped by cultural and political contingencies unique to particular countries.[7] The resilience of psychoanalysis in France, for example, is partly due to the influence of Jacques Lacan (1901–1981), but also a product of a French intellectual tradition that has privileged freedom of thought over rigid biological determinism.[8] As a result, autism is often seen in psychoanalytical terms in France, despite the fact that psychiatrists in most other countries interpret it as a neurological disorder.[9]

There can also be significant regional, as well as national, discrepancies. Although hyperactivity is seen as an American disorder, that does not mean that it is evenly distributed across the US. Statistics from the Centers for Disease Control and Prevention (CDC) indicate that diagnostic rates vary widely from state to state, ranging from 5.6 per cent prevalence in Nevada to 15.6 per cent in North Carolina.[10] The reasons for such a wide discrepancy could include the presence and activity of hyperactivity support groups, such as Children and Adults with ADD (CHADD), the philosophy and procedures of regional educational boards with respect to identifying the disorder, the degree to which the disorder is screened for by local health authorities, the marketing strategies of pharmaceutical companies and the variances in how different ethnic groups view hyperactivity and are seen as hyperactive. Similarly, although the Brazilian study above reflects that country's increasingly biomedical approach to hyperactivity, there are some areas in Brazil that have fervently resisted such developments.[11] As an increasing amount of medical history and anthropology is now beginning to show, local differences are often the key to explaining and understanding variances in experiences of health and illness.[12]

Despite regional variations, an underlying trend can also be identified which helps to explain the international proliferation of hyperactivity. Specifically, hyperactivity can be seen as an example of medical globalization at work. Medical globalization is characterized by many features, including: the incorporation or infiltration of non-Western medical traditions (Ayurvedic, Chinese) into Western medicine and the process in reverse; the predominance of market forces in health provision; global health epidemics and responses; health tourism; international medical training; and the instantaneous spread of ideas about health through the Internet.[13] Such thinking is also reflected in journalist Ethan Watters's *Crazy Like Us: The Globalization of the Western Mind*, which demonstrates that hyperactivity is not the only American disorder to go global. Focusing on anorexia in Hong Kong, PTSD in Sri Lanka, schizophrenia in Zanzibar and depression in Japan, Watters argues that the understanding of the mind in many corners of the globe has been Americanized, primarily to suit the profit motives of pharmaceutical companies.[14]

Watters's indictment of the pharmaceutical industry is certainly relevant in the case of hyperactivity, but other factors are also important to consider, as he, too, concedes. Among the most important has been the spread of a particularly Western medical notion, namely, the universalism and essentialism of disorders such as hyperactivity.[15] Hyperactivity is seen to be a universal disorder in that it is thought to exist everywhere, a feature certainly stressed in the Brazilian research and indicated by the emergence of the ADHD World Federation. Its essentialism is reflected in the notion that, wherever hyperactivity is found, it will be characterized by the same key features, course of progression and outcomes.[16] Since a hyperactive child in Africa is afflicted by the same neurological dysfunction, he should be diagnosed using the same guidelines and treated using the same drugs as a child in North America, regardless of the fact that the social, educational, cultural, domestic and environmental experiences of each child might be completely different. According to psychiatrists Sami Timimi and Begum Maitra, the application of this 'narrow deterministic biomedical template' to hyperactivity has contributed to the international spread of the disorder, despite 'the differing beliefs and practices which exist and change over time and across cultural groups with regard to the nature of childhood and child rearing'.[17] Instead of being fundamental to any understanding of childhood behaviour, the cultural dimension has been ignored in the drive to validate the universal and essential nature of hyperactivity.

Although the potency of universalism and essentialism in terms of conceptualizing mental illness has been considerable and will continue to influence how hyperactivity is understood and experienced throughout the world, it is important not to underestimate the power of local factors, rooted in culture, history and politics, to challenge such ideas. The case studies provided below indicate how universal and essential notions of hyperactivity have been both accepted and questioned in different national contexts, often in surprising ways. As with all other aspects of hyperactivity and its history, the closer one examines the conditions in which it flourishes, the less it appears to be a universal, fixed glitch in neurological functioning, present in 5.29 per cent of the human population, and the more it becomes a product of culture.

Sleeping with an Elephant – Hyperactivity in Canada

During a speech to the Press Club in Washington, DC, in 1969, less than a year after he became prime minister of Canada, Pierre Trudeau (1919–2000) described how Canada's juxtaposition with the US was 'like sleeping with an elephant. No matter how friendly and even-tempered is the beast, if I can call it that, one is affected by every twitch and grunt'.[18] Although the famous lines might help to explain the prickly relationship between the liberal Trudeau and President Richard Nixon, and have been applied to everything from Canadian economic, foreign, trade and environmental policy to the vicissitudes of the Canadian Football League, they have an ambiguity when it comes to Canadian experiences and provision of health-care. On the one hand, the proximity of the 'Darwinian US health care system', characterized by private insurance and unequal access to services, with nearly 44 million Americans (almost 15 per cent) lacking health insurance, has compelled Canadians to place a high value on their own public health care system, established in 1966.[19] Canadian fondness for Medicare, the unofficial name for the health system, was not only reflected in a recent poll which found that 86 per cent of Canadians preferred their health system to that of their American neighbours, but was also demonstrated in a 2004 television programme when Tommy Douglas (1904–1986), known as the father of Medicare, was voted the 'Greatest Canadian'.[20] Medicare has been among the most crucial factors in shaping Canada's national identity during the last 50 years, especially in terms of distinguishing the country from its southern neighbour.

Medical practice in Canada (as opposed to provision), on the other hand, has long been influenced by American medical traditions. Regardless of who eventually foots the bill, medical education, clinical practice, professional administration and medical knowledge in Canada and the US have developed along similar lines. Both Canadian and American medical schools, for example, were the subject of Abraham Flexner's (1866–1959) report on medical education, and medical programmes in both countries followed his recommendations after they were published in 1910.[21] Although William Osler (1849–1919) remains the most famous example of a physician who thrived in both Canada and the US, countless other physicians have worked in both countries, with Canadians holding administrative positions in American medical associations and vice versa. Perhaps the most telling example of the elephantine effect American medicine has had on Canadian physicians is the Canadian Medical Association's continual interest in adding elements of privatization to the Canadian health care system, despite the popularity of Medicare.[22]

Generally speaking, understandings and treatment of hyperactivity in Canada have both mirrored and influenced developments in the US, although the disorder did take longer to take hold north of the border. Given all of the ties with the US, particularly in terms of medical knowledge and exposure to American media, it is somewhat surprising that the disorder was not recognized very soon after its emergence in the US. The political and educational climate, however, so important in setting the stage for creating the alarm about hyperactivity in the US, was never as fervent in Canada during the late 1950s and early 1960s. The Canadian media began to write stories about hyperactivity as a disorder in the early 1970s, but journalists were as likely to describe hyperactivity as a normal feature of childhood, particularly among younger children.[23] In 1968, an article in *Canadian Family Physician* similarly discussed aggressive, impulsive, spontaneous and delinquent behaviour in adolescents, but not in terms of a distinct disorder such as hyperactivity. Amphetamines were mentioned, but only with respect to their use in depression, which was discouraged by the author.[24] A year later, however, an article on drugs and child psychiatry did discuss the use of amphetamines in the treatment of hyperactivity, stating that such drugs could 'cause a rapid and amazing change, the child becoming calmer, much less active and amenable to teaching'.[25] Soon hyperactivity was being discussed in other Canadian medical journals, and in the Canadian media, as regularly as those published in the US.

The growing Canadian interest in hyperactivity, however, did not mean that Canadian researchers simply aped their American colleagues in terms of how to approach the disorder. On the contrary, a number of Canadian researchers became influential players in shaping the way in which hyperactivity would be understood both in

Canada and the US. Particularly important was a team of researchers in Montreal who, starting in the mid-1960s, began to investigate hyperactivity from a number of perspectives, contributing especially to the expansion of the disorder in terms of its clinical symptoms, its medical treatment and its geographical and chronological scope.[26] Although their initial research helped to convince clinicians of the efficacy of stimulants, subsequent work on the disorder in Montreal also spurred the medical community to see hyperactivity as a lifelong disorder, a condition that affected children worldwide and a dysfunction that had inattention, as well as hyperactivity, at its core. In this way, the Montreal team helped to fashion hyperactivity as a disorder that could persist into adulthood and afflicted not only overactive boys, but also girls whose symptoms of inattention were believed to be overlooked. Despite being central to these developments, which would contribute enormously to the perceived hyperactivity epidemic, the overall approach of the Montreal team to hyperactivity, and of Canadian physicians more generally, tended to be more cautious, more holistic and more nuanced than that of their American neighbours.

Working out of McGill University and the Montreal Children's Hospital, the team, whose members included Virginia Douglas, Gabrielle Weiss, Klaus Minde, Lily Hechtman and John Werry, and whose research was often funded by pharmaceutical companies, initially encountered resistance to their biological approach. As Weiss explained in a recent interview, the Psychiatry Department at the Hospital 'had a strong psychoanalytic orientation' and employed play therapy as their primary treatment modality. Weiss and her fellow resident, New Zealander John S. Werry, were assigned to observe the play therapy sessions, but

> hyperactive boys were not good at playing quietly, allowing the therapist to 'interpret' their play. Instead they would run out of the playroom on the fifth floor on to the elevator and press the button for the twelfth floor. The therapist would follow but by the time he reached the twelfth floor the boy would be back on the fifth. As a result of failing to benefit from play therapy there were no other treatments available

so almost one hundred hyperactive boys were left and no one knew how to help them.[27]

Despite the hesitation of the Department, Weiss and Werry began a series of trials testing the efficacy of various psychoactive drugs on such children. The studies revealed that, while the antipsychotic Chlorpromazine was ineffective, the amphetamine Dexedrine successfully reduced the hyperactivity of their subjects and helped them to concentrate better.[28] Such findings were in accordance with those of American studies, particularly those done by Eisenberg and Conners, and provided additional evidence for psychiatrists, and pharmaceutical companies, keen to promote the use of stimulants in hyperactive children.

Although Werry returned to New Zealand, where he would continue to be a prominent proponent of stimulant therapy for hyperactivity, Weiss and her colleagues would continue to monitor the progress of the children, who were mainly boys, during their childhood, adolescence and adulthood, one of the first long-term follow-up studies in the field.[29] One of the major questions facing hyperactivity researchers during the 1960s was whether or not the symptoms of the disorder would diminish as the child grew into adolescence. Although opinions varied, most psychiatrists believed that the behaviour of hyperactive children would improve, suggesting that there was a developmental component to the disorder. The Montreal group sought to test this assumption by comparing how their group fared academically, vocationally, cognitively, emotionally and socially with a control group over many years, assessing them using everything from self-esteem checklists to electroencephalograms.[30] Reflecting on the results of the longitudinal studies, Weiss observed that, though both the control and the hyperactive group had their share of problems, the members of the hyperactive group had more trouble coping with life's hardships, and that these difficulties often persisted into adulthood and developed into more serious psychiatric problems.[31] These findings helped to convince the medical community that hyperactivity was not merely developmental, but existed as an adult disorder, thus contributing to increasing numbers of adults being diagnosed with hyperactivity. It also put pressure on educators and physicians to identify hyperactivity as a possible predictor for subsequent academic failure and mental illness.

Such findings could be seen as an enormous boon to drug companies, who could begin recommending that stimulants be prescribed to adults as well as children, but, according to Weiss, the situation was more complicated than that. Despite her team's initially positive findings regarding stimulants, Weiss admitted that, in the long term, such drugs 'did not necessarily influence the outcome [of the hyperactive subjects] which was multi-determined'.[32] Indeed, Weiss hoped that future treatment of hyperactive individuals would include psychodynamic elements and be multidisciplinary in its approach.[33] Establishing an appropriate educational and vocational setting was also important for both hyperactive children and adults. Weiss acknowledged that, while teachers often rated the hyperactive subjects worse than the control subjects, their eventual employers often found no difference, suggesting that the social environment, including a suitable vocation, was a key determinant of what types of behaviour were deemed to be problematic.[34]

Weiss's complex attitude towards hyperactivity was also reflected in other members of the Montreal team, particularly McGill psychiatrist Klaus Minde, who participated in some of Weiss's original drug trials. Minde's longstanding interest in Africa and the cultural aspects of psychiatric disorders spurred him to investigate whether or not hyperactivity was an issue in Uganda. Just as Weiss's longitudinal research was a novel approach to hyperactivity and key to lingering questions about the potential scope of the disorder globally, Minde's study was one of the first cross-cultural studies of the disorder to emerge during the 1970s, and the first to involve Africa. Although Minde and his co-author, Nancy Cohen, doubted that they would find evidence of the disorder in Uganda, they found themselves to be mistaken.[35] Ugandan children could also manifest the symptoms of hyperactivity. Nevertheless, there were key differences in how the disorder manifested itself in Canada and in Uganda. Whereas hyperactivity caused Canadian children to be impulsive, their Ugandan counterparts tended to be more aggressive and short-tempered. The authors also acknowledged that cultural differences did play a role in how concerned parents and teachers were about such behaviour. Ugandan parents, for instance, often saw such behaviour as a nuisance, rather than a medical disorder, and often children with pronounced symptoms were simply not sent to school.[36] Although such findings were used as evidence for the universality of hyperactivity, they could also be used to stress how the expression and interpretation of childhood behaviour is contingent upon cultural differences.

Similarly, Minde's comments in an editorial in 1975 indicated that, while he believed hyperactivity was rooted in genetics, the social environment played an even larger role:

> The majority of children who have difficulties with the world around them are not primarily hyperactive but are reacting to an environment that does not provide them with the necessary ingredients for their development. An understanding of these developmental needs can only be gained when we assess the total life-space of a child, which includes school, family and the child himself. . . . Children who receive little personal attention from their environment and get much of their entertainment from watching television are often bored and become restless, impulsive and aggressive. These children most often need people who they can trust, rather than drugs.[37]

Minde warned that many physicians, preoccupied with pharmacotherapy, overlooked the social and environmental aspects of hyperactivity, resulting in the over-prescription and over-dosage of drugs such as Ritalin. In this editorial, and elsewhere, Minde also commented on the difficulty in diagnosing the disorder, particularly in younger children, and stressed the importance of the psychosocial aspects of hyperactivity.[38] Such a multifaceted approach to hyperactivity was particularly rare among those who researched the disorder. Given the contentious nature of the disorder and its drug treatment, it was much more likely for medical commentators to discuss hyperactivity in much more uncompromising, if not polemical, terms, taking pains to defend the biological approach rather than acknowledge its complexity. Although Minde is justifiably well known for his work on the original drug trials and developing the notion that hyperactivity was not only a Western psychiatric disorder, his concern about the hyperactive child's social environment also highlights the subtleties often found in Canadian approaches to hyperactivity.

Similar nuances are evident in the final, most significant, way in which the Montreal team influenced how hyperactivity was to be understood. Psychologist Virginia Douglas had worked with Minde and Weiss to test the effect of various drugs on the symptoms of hyperactivity during the late 1960s. Although she would continue to investigate the psychopharmacology of hyperactivity, by the early 1970s she had also begun to question the core symptoms of the disorder. Ever since it was named hyperkinetic impulse disorder by Laufer and Denhoff, hyperactivity was characterized by, well, hyperactivity. But what drove such energetic and rambunctious behaviour? And why were boys so much more liable to be diagnosed than girls? The Montreal team, and particularly Douglas, suspected that, for many children, a deficit in attention was the underlying explanation for their hyperactive, impulsive and aggressive behaviour.[39] In other words, an inability to concentrate on tasks such as schoolwork, household chores or reading underpinned the impulsive and hyperactive outbursts that characterized such children. After conducting a series of trials, Douglas was not only convinced that inattention was the key feature in the hyperactivity of many children, but also that stimulant drugs could help such children improve their ability to focus and pay attention.[40]

The most obvious result of this shift in focus was that hyperactivity was described as Attention Deficit Disorder (ADD) in DSM-III (1980). For the first time, attention, not hyperactivity, was the key symptom and was reflected in the official terminology. Since one of the overarching themes of DSM-III was to make diagnosis of mental disorders more reliable and objective, this newfound attention to attention changed the way in which clinicians viewed the disorder, encouraging them to consider problems of inattention more seriously. Researchers similarly began to ask different questions about hyperactivity, based on the change in terminology. There were also implications for teachers and patients. In DSM-III, ADD could be present with hyperactivity (ADD-H) or without. This meant that hyperactive children need not be troublemakers, delinquents or class clowns; they could also be day-dreaming students who struggled at school but failed to cause enough disruption to be recognized as problematic, let alone pathological. ADD became a potent explanation as to why these children, who often tested highly on intelligence tests, failed to reach their potential. Although hyperactivity would re-enter the terminology in DSM-III-R (1987), with the term Attention Deficit/Hyperactivity Disorder (ADHD), the emphasis on inattention nevertheless suggested that the disorder could go unnoticed in children, and adults, for years.

The focus on inattention also had major implications for the epidemiology of hyperactivity. Specifically, it gave an answer to a conundrum that had been plaguing researchers for years – namely, if hyperactivity was a genetic disorder, why was it seen more often in boys than girls?[41] Now the answer appeared to be that girls were more often of the inattentive, rather than the hyperactive, type. Quiet, unassuming and placid, such girls would not likely be singled out as being troublesome by their teachers, but their attention deficit meant that their scholastic performance suffered regardless. As a result they tended to be under-diagnosed.[42] Such thinking rein- forced for many proponents of hyperactivity that the disorder was not over-diagnosed, but actually should be diagnosed far more often, especially in girls and boys who were of the inattentive, rather than hyperactive, type. The emphasis on attention also allowed adults, who may have outgrown their childhood hyperactivity to a certain extent, to be increasingly diagnosed. In their case, inatten- tion might manifest itself in problems both at work and in the home – for example, failing to meet deadlines, pay bills on time or pick children up from school. Overall, Douglas's stress on attention reaffirmed for many physicians that hyperactivity remained a hidden disorder that was often overlooked and under-diagnosed.

The contributions of Weiss, Minde, Douglas and their Montreal colleagues changed the way in which hyperactivity would be con- ceptualized in the medical community and made it possible for the disorder to proliferate both in North America and around the world.

In this way, it could be argued that Canadian understandings of hyperactivity shaped those held in the US even more than the reverse. But while these findings of the McGill researchers made a major impact on understandings of hyperactivity, paving the way for the disorder to be seen in more universal and essential terms, the subtle caveats made especially by Weiss and Minde about the social, cultural and environmental complexities of hyperactivity were not as influential. Most American hyperactivity researchers remained unmoved by the relatively holistic and measured approach to hyperactivity espoused by researchers such as Weiss and Minde, and reflected more generally in Canadian clinicians. Few American psychiatrists would endorse the multifaceted methods of Canadian physician Ray Holland, who wrote to the *Canadian Medical Association Journal* about hyperactivity in 1988. Holland prescribed Ritalin to one of his patients, but recommended an elimination diet to another and found that a more structured social environment was most effective in four others. He believed that the shift in terminology to ADHD had made the condition increasingly vague, led to over-diagnosis and moved the blame away from society itself, which was not structured in a way to motivate children to reach their potential.[43] Similar letters, particularly after the Canadian Paediatric Society produced a statement in 1990 that came close to encouraging the use of Ritalin in Canada, also indicated how Canadian physicians often resisted conventional approaches to hyperactivity. Such resistance to seeing hyperactivity as purely a neurological disorder that requires stimulant treatment was simply not seen as much in American journals.[44] Despite sleeping with an elephant, it was possible for Canadian researchers and clinicians to fashion a uniquely Canadian response to hyperactivity, one often shaped by typical Canadian characteristics of compromise, negotiation and multidisciplinarity.

Across the Pond: UK Resistance to Hyperactivity

Resistance to the rigid American approach to hyperactivity could also take different forms. Unlike Canadian physicians, who were relatively quick to acknowledge the existence of hyperactivity as a distinct medical disorder, the British medical community, which also had strong American connections, was hesitant to accept the concept until well into the 1990s. Despite the furore caused by hyperactivity in North America during the 1960s, it did not receive any mention from the *Lancet* until 1970, and this was merely a letter to the editor from a team of American psychiatrists.[45] The only reply to the letter was also written by an American psychiatrist.[46] Although there were occasional references to hyperactive behaviour in the *British Medical Journal* (BMJ) prior to the 1970s, most often in relation to epilepsy, brain damage and lead poisoning, the journal's first article specifically about the disorder was not published until 1968, when Philip Graham and Michael Rutter published one of their influential surveys of child psychiatric disorders on the Isle of Wight.[47] Most articles in the *British Journal of Psychiatry* (previously called the *Journal of Mental Science*) prior to the 1980s also tended to discuss hyperactivity as a symptom of underlying conditions, ranging from encephalitis to phenylketonuria, rather than as a disorder unto itself.[48] British media stories about hyperactivity were similarly rare, and those that were published tended to address the issue in North America, rather than what was happening in the UK.[49] Significant British interest in hyperactivity did not begin to match that in North America until the 1990s and 2000s, with one study of the relevant literature determining that, while there were only 356 publications on the topic between 1985 and 1989, during 2005–9 there were 6,158.[50]

There were many reasons for the initial reluctance of British physicians to recognize hyperactivity as a distinct childhood disorder. Crucially, psychiatrists in the UK were less keen to embrace the biomedical model of mental illness than their colleagues across the Atlantic. In the preface to the British edition of Schrag and Divoky's *The Myth of the Hyperactive Child*, criminologist Steven Box (1937–1987) argued that, while child psychiatry could be considered a 'growth industry' in the UK during the 1970s, there was 'a strong anti-drug therapy feeling among British child psychiatric experts'.[51] As a consultant child psychiatrist remarked to *The Times* in 1981, 'I don't practise chemical warfare against children'.[52]

One of the reasons for such antipathy towards psychopharmacology was the hesitance in the UK, epitomized by the pioneering psychiatrist Michael Rutter, to accept that mental illness was only the result of organic brain dysfunction. Unlike American psychiatrists, who had largely abandoned the tenets of social psychiatry by the mid-1970s, British psychiatrists were keen to 'ameliorate the psychosocial stresses' that contributed to childhood mental illness.[53] When Rutter compared rates of childhood mental illness on the Isle of Wight to those found in inner London, for instance, he found that the London rates were twice as high. The explanation for this, according to Rutter, was the additional stresses faced by children living in a chaotic modern metropolis, as well as those encountered by their parents.[54] Another British study found that hyperactivity was a common characteristic of maltreated children.[55] Still other British psychiatrists echoed that 'social and family factors may be the most important influences bearing on the behaviour of young children' and questioned the role played by neurological dysfunction.[56] Or, as an editorial in the Lancet asked in 1973: 'Are the Americans ahead of the British, or behind them, or do their children's brains dysfunction in such an ostentatiously exotic transatlantic fashion that they require drug therapy?'[57] The tone of the editorial suggested that the Americans might well be behind their British colleagues, or perhaps thrusting ahead towards a biological psychiatry with which many British psychiatrists would feel uncomfortable.

Another reason for the paucity of hyperactivity diagnoses was related to the terminology used to describe troublesome children in the UK. While British schoolchildren were often described by educators as 'maladjusted' or 'medium educational subnormal', British psychiatrists might diagnose them with 'conduct disorder', 'school phobia', 'emotional disorder' or even 'autism'. Such terms might have been fairly disparate in terms of the behaviour that would be exhibited by such children, but nevertheless reflected the influence of both psychoanalysis and social psychiatry in British psychiatry. Although British children diagnosed with conduct disorder might have been given a hyperactivity diagnosis had they lived in the US, the problems of these children were still seen in psychosocial, rather than biological, terms in the UK. Drugs, again unlike in the US, were rarely used as treatment.[58] When British psychiatrists did diagnose children with hyperactivity as a distinctive disorder, the symptoms were not only much more severe than those described in diagnoses of hyperactivity made in North America, but they were also associated with organic brain damage from an injury or illness.[59] In the UK, hyperactivity was not normally seen as a disorder associated with troublesome schoolchildren.

When hyperactivity was recognized as a distinct disorder, it was common for environmental causes, such as food additives, heavy metal exposure and malnutrition, as well as organic brain damage, to be singled out. Three of the British associations that advocated the legitimacy of hyperactivity during the 1970s, for example, stressed the role of environmental factors in triggering hyperactivity.[60] One of these groups, the Hyperactive Children's Support Group, founded by Sally Bunday during the late 1970s, even published a collection of their members' success stories – employing food-additive-free diets – entitled *The Proof of the Pudding*.[61] Such thinking was also reflected in many of the first articles written about the disorder in the UK, in media coverage and in the tenor of the editorials which commented on the Feingold diet during the 1970s and 1980s.[62]

As chapter Five indicates, British interest in the link between food additives and hyperactivity, emanating from both the public and the medical spheres, has persisted, reflecting both longstanding and ongoing British concern about chemicals in food and the safety of the food supply more generally. Not only have the most recent trials of additive-free diets been conducted in the UK, the Southampton trial, which was sponsored by the Food Standards Agency (FSA), was prompted by public interest in the issue. The Southampton group's positive findings generated an enormous amount of media attention, as well as an unprecedented amount of feedback directed towards the FSA, according to its chief scientist, Andrew Wadge.[63] Such a large degree of interest in the link between food additives and hyperactivity does indicate that, by the 2000s, hyperactivity was a major concern in the UK, but it also suggests that unconventional explanations and treatments for the disorder were also widespread.

Despite the interest in environmental causes and the research of psychiatrists such as Rutter and Graham, however, there was little indication of a hyperactivity epidemic in Britain during the 1980s, even after the disorder, termed 'hyperkinetic syndrome of childhood', was included in WHO's *International Classification of Diseases* (ICD-9) in 1978.[64] In 1984, an article stated that, while the disorder dominated 30–40 per cent of the clinical population seen by North American child psychiatrists, there had only been 73 hyperactive children seen at the Maudsley and Bethlem Royal Hospitals in London between 1968 and 1980.[65] There were signs, however, that concern about hyperactivity was beginning to make its way across the Atlantic. A *Lancet* editorial in 1986 concurred that 'British paediatricians, family practitioners and child psychiatrists are far less ready than their colleagues in the USA to diagnose and treat a syndrome of hyperactivity', but also cautioned that 'severe and pervasive hyperactivity is a risk factor and can handicap social development' and that 'British medicine and education will need to make its modification a higher priority'.[66] Another article by London psychiatrist Eric Taylor, who was largely responsible for promoting the diagnosis of hyperactivity in the UK, similarly suggested that both British educators and physicians should recognize hyperactivity more often, although he also suspected that the disorder was over-diagnosed in the US.[67] One of the ways in which British psychiatrists should do this, Taylor and others suggested, was by distinguishing hyperactivity from conduct disorder, which was a common diagnosis in the UK.[68] Hyperactivity had to be treated more seriously in the UK, argued psychiatrists such as Taylor, but perhaps not to the enthusiastic extent as it was in the US.

As the 1990s wore on, North American approaches to hyperactivity were increasingly finding favour in the UK. A growing number of British psychiatrists became convinced that the differential rates of hyperactivity diagnoses in the UK and the US were not a question of cultural difference, as some suspected, but were due to the diagnostic criteria they were using.[69] Much of the confusion rested on the differences between DSM and ICD measures for the disorder. The DSM criteria used by North American physicians were less stringent than those of the ICD, which were used more often in the UK. According to the National Institute for Health and Clinical Excellence (NICE), when ICD was used, only 1–2 per cent of children would be diagnosed as hyperactive; when DSM-IV was used, the rate was estimated to be 3–9 per cent.[70] Believing that the North American criteria were preferable, Eric Taylor, along with fellow psychiatrist Peter Hill, published a protocol in 2001 for dealing with hyperactivity which was based on DSM-IV criteria.[71] Using the DSM-IV criteria, a subsequent community sample estimated that 8 per cent of the childhood population presented the symptoms of the disorder – figures quite similar to estimates of its prevalence in North America.[72]

Not surprisingly, given the shift in diagnostic criteria, British rates of hyperactivity diagnoses increased considerably during the 2000s.[73] Public awareness of the disorder in the UK also grew, in part due to the emergence of hyperactivity support groups, but also because of the Internet, which such groups effectively used to attract and support members. British researchers also began embracing the notion that hyperactivity was rooted in genetics, rather than environmental or social factors, and embarked upon twin studies to demonstrate their theories.[74] Finally, British psychiatrists began prescribing stimulants at a much higher rate throughout the 1990s and 2000s, suggesting that North American approaches to hyperactivity had finally infiltrated the UK.[75]

But even as British rates of hyperactivity increased and stimulant medication became more common, significant differences remained in terms of how the disorder was perceived in the UK when compared to the US. Although official bodies such as NICE have affirmed the validity of hyperactivity as a medical condition, they have also recognized that opposing positions were justifiable and that what is defined as abnormal behaviour is driven by contemporary social views.[76] NICE has also been less confident about the causes of hyperactivity and the best ways to treat it. In a recent set of guidelines, for example, they stressed that 'The diagnosis of ADHD does not imply a medical or neurological cause. . . . The aetiology of ADHD involves the interplay of multiple genetic and environmental factors.'[77] Listed alongside genetics as possibly contributing to the disorder were environmental influences, such as exposure to lead, tobacco and alcohol, diet and psychosocial factors. The acknowledgement of such a wide range of causative factors signifies more than an appreciation of unconventional approaches to the disorder; it also underlines a realization that hyperactivity is complex, often triggered by many factors, and has to be treated as such. Accordingly, the treatment options listed in the guidelines certainly discussed medication, but also mentioned educational, behavioural, psychological, parenting and dietary interventions. Indeed, the first case study presented in the guidelines featured the story of a patient diagnosed with hyperactivity who overcame his difficulties without drugs, finding that physical exercise, creative outlets, a rewarding career and counselling were preferable.[78] NICE has argued against prescribing drugs to preschool children for hyperactivity, and only advocated medication for older children whose symptoms were severe and those with moderate symptoms who did not respond to other interventions.[79]

When compared to the American approach, which has emphasized the genetic and neurological aspects of hyperactivity and stressed the benefits of stimulant medication at the expense of other interventions, even for very young children, it is clear that British notions of hyperactivity remain less rigid, more open-ended and certainly less confident.[80] Although there are numerous physicians who espouse American-style biomedical theories of hyperactivity, there are likely just as many who are sceptical and opt for a more balanced, multifaceted view of the disorder. Even when hyperactivity is accepted as a medical diagnosis, British psychiatrists are more willing to consider alternative explanations and treatments. Medical globalization has certainly influenced the gradual emergence of hyperactivity as a legitimate and widespread psychiatric disorder in the UK, but it is apparent that British understandings and experiences of the disorder have also been shaped by a particularly British approach to psychiatry and childhood mental illness. For British psychiatrists, and for the British public, childhood behavioural problems may have genetic and neurological aspects, but these always interact with, and often pale in comparison to, the social, domestic, educational and environmental factors ever-present in the lives of children.

Despite the fact that countries such as Canada and the UK have taken steps to approach hyperactivity in their own way, it is also clear that the idea of hyperactivity as a neurological dysfunction best treated with drugs is spreading rapidly across the globe. In the last twenty years the production of methylphenidate (Ritalin) increased by a factor of sixteen and the drug is used to treat hyperactivity in 100 countries. Between 2004 and 2008 alone, global consumption of Ritalin and related drugs rose from 28.2 tonnes (31 US tons) to 52 tonnes (57 US tons) per year. Although Americans consumed 75 per cent of that amount, their share of the total has been declining. Moreover, Icelanders, not Americans, now swallow the most Ritalin tablets per capita. Although it has been suggested that the midnight sun in summer might have something to do with the prevalence of hyperactivity in northern latitudes, the fact that there is an Icelandic jazz band called ADHD also suggests, however, that the disorder is developing a cultural relevancy.[81]

Generally speaking, however, cultural awareness of hyperactivity or hyperactive children has not spread as quickly as medical awareness of the disorder or tablets of Ritalin and other drugs. There are scant international examples of Percy Jackson, the twelve-year-old hero of Rick Riordan's popular *Camp Half Blood* children's book series, whose ADHD diagnosis and dyslexia has resulted in him being expelled from countless schools. It makes perfect sense for the hero of an American children's novel to be hyperactive, given the high numbers of children diagnosed with the disorder. Such children have been a prominent part of American culture for many decades and, when the behavioural tendencies of a hyperactive child are considered from a more positive perspective, it is not surprising that such energetic, creative and assertive children make for good heroes. But where are the Chinese, Nigerian or Brazilian Percy Jacksons? It could be that it will take time for hyperactivity in the rest of the world to gain the cultural currency it has in North America. But it could also be that their absence is indicative of an artificiality to the global emergence of hyperactivity, and that American notions of childhood behaviour and stimulant therapy have been forcibly applied to children from very different backgrounds.

Pharmaceutical companies, driven primarily by commercial rather than health interests, must be considered largely responsible for pushing such ideas, along with their products.[82] Companies such as Novartis and Janssen Pharmaceuticals market both the notion of hyperactivity and the drugs that treat it across the globe, not only sponsoring the World Congresses on ADHD, but other international conferences and medical research. As a result, while the bulk of scientific literature on hyperactivity continues to emanate from the US, international researchers are closing the gap. Pharmaceutical companies have facilitated international interest by providing funding opportunities, but equally important has been the spread of the biomedical model of mental illness. The current neurological and genetic paradigm not only explains away children's behavioural problems in a neat and tidy fashion, it also allows researchers the world over to speak the same language when it comes to conceptualizing mental illness. Culturally speaking, international researchers are not so different from their American colleagues and, although the children they study may be growing up in vastly different circumstances from American children, it is assumed that their brains are identical. Since the details of how hyperactive children's brains function (or dysfunction, perhaps) and the mechanism of stimulant drugs remain tantalizingly elusive, it is possible to build long-term research programmes, funded by pharmaceutical companies, to explore these and other puzzles, all the while reaffirming the existence of hyperactivity as a biological reality. One's country of birth or mother tongue may not be a barrier to such endeavours, but a wavering belief in the biomedical model is. Those who do not speak the biomedical language, as a recent history of autism demonstrates, are shunned and ridiculed as unscientific dinosaurs.[83]

Underlying such developments may be globalization itself and the values it upholds. Psychiatrist Sami Timimi has associated the entrenchment of free-market capitalism in the Western world and the accompanying glorification of narcissistic self-love with the proliferation of disorders such as hyperactivity, resulting in a 'McDonaldization' of children's mental health. As with fast food, the biomedical approach to childhood misbehaviour

feeds on the desire for instant satisfaction, it fits into consumers' busy lifestyles, it requires little engagement with
the product from the consumer, it requires only the most
superficial training, knowledge and understanding to produce, it de-skills people by providing an 'easy way out' . . .
it creates potentially life-long consumers for the product,
and it has the potential to produce long-term damage to
both the individuals who consume these products as well
as public health more generally.[84]

Timimi proceeds to link the economic and social insecurities of neo-
liberalism, starkly realized during the recent global recession, not
only to mental health problems in children, but also to medicine's
focus on the flawed individual, rather than the possibly pathogenic
society blamed by the social psychiatrists of the 1960s. Struggling to
compete in a uncompromising world of diminishing returns, it is
not surprising that people from China to Chile have increasingly
seen hyperactivity and its chemical cures as an explanation and
potential solution for their difficulties.

But despite the powerful influence of biomedical models,
pharmaceutical company funding and overarching neo-liberalism,
the examples of Canada and the UK, the two countries closest to
the US in terms of culture, ideology, educational methods and
medical practice, suggest that the proliferation of hyperactivity is
far more complicated and textured than the metaphor of a carbon-
copied Big Mac would suggest. If anything, the histories of
hyperactivity in Canada and the UK suggest that it is important for
both historians and medical researchers not to overgeneralize. The
5.29 per cent prevalence rate now touted emphatically by hyperactivity's promoters glosses over spectacularly the differences in
how the disorder has been understood and experienced from
country to country. In each example of how hyperactivity has been
embraced, rejected or transformed, there is a particular story that
explains why this has been the case. As Timimi and Maitra rightly
contend, cultural differences, particularly in terms of how
childhood is perceived, are at the heart of these often idiosyncratic
stories.[85]

Chinese psychiatrists, for instance, have recognized hyper-activity as being prevalent in the childhood population for decades.[86] Such interest is possibly due to the high degree of importance placed on academic success in China as well as less tolerance of disruptive behaviour.[87] But since parents, and some physicians, are often apprehensive about drug treatment, traditional Chinese medicine is often preferred.[88] Drug treatments are also viewed with suspicion in India, where hyperactivity has been less eagerly taken up.[89] In one study of resistance to hyperactivity medication in India, over 83 per cent of the subjects refused to adhere to their prescriptions. The reasons provided for this recalcitrance included side effects, inefficacy, fears that the drugs would lead to addiction, cost and the 'careless attitude of caregivers'.[90] Other researchers, however, found that the Indian parents they surveyed were reluctant to accept biomedical explanations for their children's hyperactivity, preferring instead to blame psychological, educational, social or parenting problems. Instead of opting for drugs, these parents tended to rely on educational or religious interventions. The researchers concluded, probably to the chagrin of pharmaceutical companies keen to break the vast Indian market, that 'locally acceptable illness models' need to be employed in order to help parents of children with behavioural problems in developing countries.[91] One other aspect of focusing on local conditions which is reflected in Indian hyperactivity research is a concerted interest in identifying the environmental (particularly lead pollution) and nutritional (for instance, mineral and vitamin deficiencies) causes of the disorder. Perhaps those keen to export Western notions of hyperactivity to the developing world should first focus on addressing these issues of environmental and nutritional inequality.

Local circumstances have also shaped notions of hyperactivity elsewhere. In many parts of Europe, rates of hyperactivity and stimulant prescriptions have increased enormously, but when one examines how the disorder has been dealt with in specific countries, fascinating and contradictory stories emerge. Within the Nordic countries alone, use of hyperactivity drugs varies considerably. Children in Iceland are ten times more likely to be prescribed drugs than their counterparts in Finland, where hyperactivity is seen as more of an 'everyday educational challenge' rather than a pathology.[92] In Sweden, the history of hyperactivity has been shaped by two developments: the government's decision in 1968 to ban Ritalin, due to reports of its abuse, and more recently the so-called Gillberg Affair, involving prominent child psychiatrist Christopher Gillberg. The affair might have been sparked by Gillberg's decision to shred tens of thousands of documents relating to a longitudinal study of severely hyperactive children, but chiefly involved the prevalence and causes of childhood psychiatric disorders such as hyperactivity.[93] While Gillberg believed that 10 per cent of Swedish children suffered from neuropsychiatric disorder, this was disputed by academics Leif Elinder and Eva Kärvfe, who published a book in 2000 that strongly contradicted Gillberg's claims. Gillberg was outraged and accused Elinder and Kärvfe of basing their arguments on documents supplied by the Scientology movement, which was opposed to psychopharmacology. Elinder and Kärvfe replied by accusing Gillberg of fraudulently manipulating the data from the longitudinal study and demanded to see the evidence for themselves. The request was refused and court action ensued, with the courts ruling that Elinder and Kärvfe were entitled to view Gillberg's data, despite the psychiatrist's claims that this would breach confidentiality agreements. Before they could do so, however, Gillberg had the material destroyed in 2004, resulting in fines and conditional sentences for the psychiatrist and his collaborators.

The Gillberg episode divided the Swedish scientific community, with some accusing Gillberg of being an agent for the pharmaceutical industry and others claiming that Elinder and Kärvfe had connections with Scientology. It is safe to say that neither side escaped unscathed nor acted with impunity. Moreover, the vitriol generated by the affair will undoubtedly cast a shadow on any discussion of hyperactivity in Sweden for quite some time, demonstrating how polemical attitudes continue to affect how childhood behaviour is understood.

Not every country will have its Gillberg affair. But local circumstances have undoubtedly shaped how individual countries have perceived the emergence of hyperactivity as a potent explanation for childhood behavioural problems. When the individual cases are examined in detail, it does not take long to realize that the over-arching statements made about the global prevalence and signifi-cance of hyperactivity are essentially meaningless, and generated purely to support the notion that the disorder is an essential and universal neurological dysfunction that has always existed in all times and places. Such ideas might be accepted in many countries, certainly boosting the profits of pharmaceutical companies in the process, but that does not mean they truly match how hyperactivity has been understood and experienced in countries with disparate beliefs about childhood, education, mental illness and psycho-pharmacology. Uncovering the distinct histories of hyperactivity in various countries may be one way of overturning such vapid generalizations.

Conclusion: Happily Hyperactive?

Hyperactivity is no longer just for kids. Building on the work of Gabrielle Weiss and others, and responding to emerging disability legislation, such as the US's Individuals with Disabilities Education Act (1990), psychiatrists began diagnosing adults with the disorder during the 1990s.[1] Whereas children with hyperactivity might struggle in school, adults would have difficulty at work, in their relationships and with managing their affairs. For Chuck Pearson, described in 1994 in a *Time* magazine article, hyperactivity helped to explain why he had been fired from fifteen jobs in twelve years, why he had bill collectors constantly knocking at his door and why he lost his driver's licence after forgetting to pay his parking tickets. As with many people diagnosed with hyperactivity as adults, Pearson, who self-medicated with 30–40 cups of coffee per day, was diagnosed following the diagnosis of one of his children. Feeling 'a deep and abiding sadness over the life I could have given my family if I had been treated effectively', Pearson founded the Adult Attention Deficit Foundation, which offers information about the disorder.[2] When 43-year-old gym teacher and entrepreneur Karenne Bloomgarden, also described in the article, was told by her doctor that she had hyperactivity, it was both a revelation and a relief: 'I had 38 years of thinking I was a bad person. Now I'm rewriting the tapes of who I thought I was to who I really am.'[3]

For others, the impact of a hyperactivity diagnosis and the resultant stimulant medication was less profound, but still positive. Helen, a 43-year-old mother of three, was finally able 'to sit down and listen to what my husband had done at work'. She was now able to 'sit in bed and read while my husband watched TV'.[4]

Despite these stories, and the interviews of numerous proponents of the disorder, the overall tone of the article was circumspect. The authors noted how 'ADHD awareness has become an industry, a passion, an almost messianic movement', fuelled in part by support groups like CHADD and self-help books. They also stressed that, while drugs could be beneficial, both hyperactive children and adults also benefited from suitable environments, whether that meant desks at which schoolchildren could stand, rather than sit, or adults selecting careers where their hyperactive tendencies could work to their advantage. Bruce Roseman, for example, a neurologist whose work environment allowed him to be creative and leave bookkeeping and organizational details to others, felt that his hyperactivity aided him in his work, declaring: 'Thank God for my add [sic].'[5] But what about those who were unable to find a career that matched their strengths? Conformist American society, the article contended, where a college degree was a necessary condition of success, had created a situation in which 'it was necessary to medicate some people to make them fit in'. What was needed instead was 'a society that was more flexible in its expectations, more accommodating to differences'.[6]

Two decades later, there are still no simple answers about hyperactivity, what it represents about children (and adults) and the societies in which they live. A seemingly infinite number of disparate views and opinions continue to abound. In the same month as the FDA reconsidered the link between food additives and hyperactivity, for example, a 2011 *Time* article suggested that many adults diagnosed with the disorder were actually malingerers. Under the heading, 'Faking it', the story commented on research which found that adult patients exaggerated their symptoms either to get a diagnosis of ADHD, which might result in academic accommodations, or to be prescribed hyperactivity drugs, widely seen as study aids.[7] According to the researchers, 'it is quite easy to feign ADHD symptoms . . . symptoms of ADHD are widely publicized in the popular press and on the internet'.[8] Such findings also accorded with an MSNBC.com poll, which found that 38 per cent of the primary care physicians surveyed suspected that their patients also exaggerated symptoms to get diagnosed with the disorder.[9] At the root of the problem, commented a neurology professor, was the 'big cultural pressure to get these drugs . . . because everyone is in an arms race of accomplishment'.[10] A BBC investigative report similarly claimed that unscrupulous parents sought ADHD diagnoses for their children in order to claim disability benefits.[11]

A Canadian documentary, entitled ADD & Loving It?!, and accompanying website featuring iconic comedians Rick Green and Patrick McKenna, themselves diagnosed with the disorder, offered the opposite assessment. Hyperactivity was not a biomedical version of 'the dog ate my homework' or a means to benefits, academic accommodations and drugs, but a potent explanation for years of frustration, failure and even habitually losing one's car keys.[12] For McKenna and Green there was nothing wrong with helping people to succeed by giving them a diagnosis that allowed them to conceptualize their behaviour in more positive ways, attempt to find environments in which their personal characteristics can be seen as strengths and, possibly, even give them access to drugs that 'level the playing field'.[13] Their website, totallyadd.com, offers the views of hyperactivity experts, dispels 'myths' about the disorder via dozens of videos (some sponsored by drug companies), provides support and even hosts a 'virtual test' to help visitors determine whether or not they might be 'totally ADD' themselves.

Views on what hyperactivity implies about children and their parents are similarly divisive. On the one hand Lisa Loomer's recent play Distracted puts the blame for the epidemic on an overload of media stimuli that, among other things, prevents parents from giving enough attention to their children.[14] On the other hand, journalist Judith Warner argues in We've Got Issues: Children and Parents in the Age of Medication that many children who do need drugs for disorders such as hyperactivity go without and suffer as a consequence.[15] From a completely different viewpoint, it could be that the multitasking required in the 'hyper-connected' world of text messaging, social networking and mobile devices are custom-designed for hyperactive children used to emailing, watching television and talking to friends on the phone all at once.[16]

Histories of hyperactivity, or at least this one, cannot reconcile all of these multifarious perspectives. But they can provide the sort of insight and context that can help not only physicians, policy makers and educators, but more importantly, patients and their families make more informed choices about how to conceptualize, explain and, possibly, change their behaviours. I have argued that it is impossible to extricate hyperactivity from the historical period in which it emerged. Neither physicians, nor society in general, were particularly concerned about overactive, impulsive and distractible children prior to the late 1950s. Hyperactive children were identified occasionally as being problematic, but when this happened, their behaviour was far more disturbing than that exhibited by hyperactive children today, often to the point that they were institutionalized. Moreover, it was usually clear that they were suffering from organic brain damage, from injury or infections, such as encephalitis, or allergies. The crucial question, therefore, becomes why did physicians begin to diagnose hyperactivity in children who were not so disturbed?

The answers that emerge involve not only changes in the labels used to describe such children, but also broad political forces emanating from Cold War tensions, demographic challenges, questions about the education system and concerns about the ability of American children to compete with their Soviet counterparts in a nuclear world. Similarly, the reasons why the disorder came to be seen in such simplistic biological terms, with little or no consideration of how aspects of a child's domestic, social and physical environment might affect his or her mental health, also transcend mere medicine. Psychiatric ambitions, corporate avarice and biomedical ideologies have also played a key role in transforming a disorder that could be conceptualized in many ways into a neurological condition best treated with stimulants. Any attempts to provide alternative explanations, whether they have focused on lead poisoning, food additives, too much television or lack of exercise, have struggled to achieve legitimacy in the face of a biopharmaceutical paradigm that is both philosophically and economically potent and now spreading across the globe. Nevertheless, the more the notion of hyperactivity migrates, the more it becomes clear that local circumstances, traditions and philosophies will in turn play an important role in changing the way the disorder is understood, experienced and perceived. Despite the best efforts of pharmaceutical companies to sell the idea of hyperactivity around the world, ultimately the decisions about whether or not a child's behaviour constitutes a medical disorder will be made in a broader context that encompasses the expectations and attitudes of very different cultures and societies.

So, what does this all mean for hyperactive children and their parents? Well, if anything, it highlights that hyperactivity, as a medical idea, is very much a product of very specific times, places and circumstances. It is not an essential and universal medical truth that is forever constant and unchanging. It is, instead, an idea that has fluctuated considerably over time and across space and will continue to do so, just as expectations of, and attitudes towards, children change. For children and parents who are confronted by the educational and medical establishment with the prospect of a hyperactivity diagnosis, the history of the disorder can be an empowering tool that allows them to accept, amend or reject such judgements with more confidence.

When other aspects of the history of hyperactivity are explored in more detail, perhaps using oral history techniques in particular, further insight can be realized. Gender, for example, would be an ideal lens through which to interpret the emergence of hyperactivity.[17] Why do boys continue to receive more diagnoses of hyperactivity than girls? How and why have expectations of boys' behaviour changed in the last few decades? Gender and education research is beginning to turn its gaze to boys rather than girls, partly because of concerns that boys are falling behind girls academically, but how has the experience of being a boy changed and has this contributed to the pathologization of boyish behaviour?[18]

Similarly, the history of children's physical activity might also have a bearing on how we understand hyperactivity. Recent research has suggested that hyperactivity is often associated with obesity in both children and adults.[19] Although researchers have tended to hypothesize that some 'fundamental biologic link' between the metabolic and cognitive systems underlies the connection, a simpler explanation could be a reduction in the amount of exercise and activity undertaken by children. Schools in the Canadian provinces of New Brunswick and Saskatchewan, according to a CBC (Canadian Broadcasting Corporation) report, have employed treadmills and other exercise equipment in the classroom in order to help students focus.[20] Although most of the comments on the CBC story were positive and enthused about also situating such equipment where adults work, one reader sarcastically added: 'Wow, it's almost as if humans weren't designed to spend 8 hours a day sitting at a small desk in a crowded room listening to an apathetic teacher/ performing menial tasks.'

To others, however, installing exercise equipment is not seeing the forest for the trees. Journalist Richard Louv argues that children suffer from 'nature deficit disorder', a condition resulting in behavioural and attention problems. The reason children lack exposure to the great outdoors, according to Louv, is a combination of parental fear of the wilderness and the unknown, limited access to natural areas and competing sedentary and indoor leisure activities.[21] Environmental scientist Michael Depledge, who served as chief scientific advisor to the UK's Environment Agency, has also linked access to nature with emotional well-being. His concept of the 'blue gym' posits that children and adults can improve their physical and mental health by getting involved in activities in or around aquatic environments.[22] One of Depledge's goals is to provide scientific evidence that can convince policy makers that such a link is valid and that initiatives like the blue gym are cost-effective ways of preventing mental and physical illness. A detailed historical survey of how children's access to exercise and nature has changed since the post-war period, taking into consideration migration to the suburbs, the rise of car culture and the proliferation of television, video games and internet entertainment, could also help to determine the validity of such instinctive notions about what affects child behaviour and learning.

Finally, the history of hyperactivity should be viewed in the context of changes in the relationship between children and the adults in their lives, primarily parents and teachers. It is not so long ago that the interactions between adults and children were moderated by the threat of physical violence; parents and teachers could effectively beat hyperactive children into docile submission.[23] During my school days, the threat of 'the strap', however judicious its use was, certainly kept me in line most of the time. Although when such corporal punishment is employed today it is widely seen as physical abuse, and justifiably so, it is possible that because of this the balance in the relationship between children and adults has shifted somewhat. Perhaps disorders such as hyperactivity have emerged in part to redress that balance, helping adults to control children biochemically, rather than physically, much like antipsychotic drugs such as Thorazine were seen as chemical straitjackets. By interpreting hyperactivity in terms of its relationship to changes in how gender expectations, physical activity and adult–child relationships, to list but three examples, have changed over time, it will be possible to develop an even more sophisticated, informed and ultimately empowering conception of it and its role in modern societies.

History has a vital role in shaping our understanding of health and illness, but in a broader sense its most important function is to lend perspective. Debates about hyperactivity may have pervaded discussions of childhood, education, psychiatry and pharmacology for 50 years, but that does not mean that the disorder will always be so clinically and culturally ubiquitous. Just as many previously prevalent mental illnesses, such as hysteria, multiple personality disorder or sexual inversion have either fallen out of fashion, been reconceptualized or been discarded completely, notions of hyperactivity and childhood behaviour will continue to shift and mutate, perhaps falling apart altogether at some point in the future. But while this means historians should be wary of making daft prognostications, it does not mean that we should shy away from not only informing but also contributing to public debates about the subjects we research.

I began this conclusion discussing hyperactivity in adults because I believe that, despite claims about its universality and essentiality, which are seen to transcend age, as well as gender, culture, ethnicity and every other social category, the disorder and its pharmaceutical treatment represent something quite different for adults as opposed to for children. Adults, to varying degrees, are responsible for their own actions and choices. If they see hyperactivity as a diagnosis that helps them understand themselves better and cope more effectively with what is a competitive and unforgiving world, then that is largely their prerogative. If they wish to take drugs to help 'level the playing field', or give themselves an edge, that is also understandable. Certainly, the rise of cosmetic surgery suggests that people are altogether too willing to put their bodies at risk in the hopes of carving out a better future for, or image of, themselves.[24] Taking a pill that helps one concentrate better seems rather benign in comparison to enlarging, shrinking, sculpting or doing anything surgical to one's body for little reason apart from vanity. The fact that we live in a society in which adults feel compelled to employ such measures, be they surgical or chemical, in order to get ahead is rather sad, but it is not altogether surprising. Perhaps Ritalin could be seen as the academic or vocational equivalent of steroids, another drug category that found favour during the late 1950s, and as a result might be perceived as cheating in some circumstances – but it might be said that if adults wish to risk using them it is largely up to them.[25]

Once children who have been diagnosed with hyperactivity become adults, it similarly becomes much easier for them to accept or reject the diagnosis. One recent instance of this involved seven-foot-tall Chris Kaman (b. 1982), a centre for the NBA's Los Angeles Clippers who grew up in Michigan. Kaman had been diagnosed with hyperactivity at the age of two, and had taken Ritalin and Adderall for many years. Described as an 'intelligent, but rambunctious youth', Kaman struggled to memorize the plays his coaches would call during basketball games, but did not feel that the medication helped.[26] In addition, the drugs sapped his appetite, making it difficult to gain the muscle mass and strength that basketball centres require. As an adult, Kaman sought a second opinion and eventually found a physician who diagnosed him with an anxiety disorder and prescribed neurofeedback therapy, training his brain to slow down his thought processes and deal with the stresses of playing professional basketball more effectively. The therapy worked and Kaman's on-court awareness and ability to follow plays improved considerably. While it could be argued that

Kaman simply replaced one biomedical disorder for another, the more important point is that, as an adult, and one with the financial resources to seek out as many second opinions as he liked, the ultimate decision in the matter was his, not his parents', his teachers' or his physician's.

For children the situation is very different. Children lack the power to contest decisions made by adults about their mental state and how to alter it. It may be that some children are simply uncontrollable in some situations and require medication from time to time. But if the history of hyperactivity can provide any insight at all, it is that such behaviour has only been seen to be disruptive in certain circumstances, typically when children are required to act less like children and more like adults. When a child's behaviour has been perceived to be pathological, the history of hyperactivity demonstrates that a countless array of factors, ranging from his or her domestic, social, cultural and educational environment to what he or she has for breakfast (if anything), have been thought to be responsible. Before adults decide to employ the easy way out, blaming genetics and offering a pill, perhaps they owe it to children to look to history and consider all of these factors first.

References

Introduction: Why the Hype?

1 Guilherme Polanczyk, Maurício Silva de Lima, Bernardo Lessa Horta, Joseph Biederman and Luis Augusto Rohde, 'The Worldwide Prevalence of ADHD: A Systematic Review and Metaregression Analysis', *American Journal of Psychiatry*, 164 (2007), pp. 942–8.

2 Anita Thapar quoted in Jane Dreaper, 'New Study Claims "ADHD has a Genetic Link"', BBC News (30 September 2010), at www.bbc.co.uk, accessed 1 October 2010.

3 Oliver James quoted in Dreaper, 'New Study Claims'.

4 Fergus Walsh, 'The Genetics of ADHD', BBC News (30 September 2010), at www.bbc.co.uk, accessed 1 October 2010.

5 It is ironic that Anderson called hyperactivity minimal brain damage since she claimed that the disorder was rooted in genetics.

6 Camilla Anderson, *Society Pays the High Cost of Minimal Brain Damage in America* (New York, 1972), pp. 214–16, 219.

7 Peter Schrag and Diane Divoky, *The Myth of the Hyperactive Child: And Other Means of Child Control* (New York, [1975] 1982), p. 37.

8 Ibid.

9 Peter Breggin, *Talking Back to Ritalin: What Doctors Aren't Telling You about Stimulants for Children* (Monroe, ME, 1998), pp. 147, 179.

10 Stephen W. Garber, Marianne Daniels Garber and Robyn Freedman Spizman, *Beyond Ritalin: Facts about Medication and Other Strategies for Helping Children, Adolescents, and Adults with Attention Deficit Disorder* (New York, 1996), p. 5.

11 Gabor Maté, *Scattered Minds: A New Look at the Origins and Healing of Attention Deficit Disorder* (Toronto, 1999); Ben F. Feingold, *Why Your*

Child is Hyperactive (New York, 1974); Matthew Smith, An Alternative History of Hyperactivity: Food Additives and the Feingold Diet (New Brunswick, NJ, 2011).

12 Nancy L. Morse, Attention Deficit Disorder: Natural Alternatives to Drug Therapy (Vancouver, 2000).

13 Richard DeGrandpre, Ritalin Nation: Rapid-fire Culture and the Transformation of Human Consciousness (New York, 1999), p. 9.

14 Thom Hartmann, Attention Deficit Disorder: A Different Perception (Grass Valley, CA, 1997).

15 David Healy, The Antidepressant Era (Cambridge, MA, 1997).

16 Mark Jackson, The Borderland of Imbecility: Medicine, Society and the Fabrication of the Feeble Mind in Late Victorian and Edwardian England (Manchester, 2000).

17 Allan Young, The Harmony of Illusions: Inventing Post-traumatic Stress Disorder (Princeton, NJ, 1995).

18 Ali Haggett, Desperate Housewives, Neuroses and the Domestic Environment, 1945–1970 (London, 2012).

19 Erika Dyck, Psychedelic Psychiatry: LSD from Clinic to Campus (Baltimore, MD, 2008); Jack D. Pressman, Last Resort: Psychosurgery and the Limits of Medicine (Cambridge, 1998).

20 Maurice W. Laufer, Eric Denhoff and Gerald Solomons, 'Hyperkinetic Impulse Disorder in Children's Behavior Problems', Psychosomatic Medicine, 19 (1957), pp. 38–49; Maurice W. Laufer and Eric Denhoff, 'Hyperkinetic Behavior Syndrome in Children', Journal of Pediatrics, 50 (1957), pp. 463–7.

21 Charles A. Malone, 'Some Observations on Children of Disorganized Families and Problems of Acting Out', Journal of the American Academy of Child Psychiatry, 2 (1963), pp. 22–49.

22 National Institute of Mental Health, 'Attention Deficit Hyperactivity Disorder among Children', at www.nimh.nih.gov, accessed 14 December 2010.

23 Perri Klass, 'Untangling the Myths about Attention Deficit Hyperactivity Disorder', New York Times (13 December 2010), at www. nytimes.com, accessed 16 December 2010.

ONE: Before Hyperactivity

1 One good recent example of this is: Klaus W. Lange, Susanne Reichl, Katharina M. Lange, Lara Tucha and Oliver Tucha, 'The History of Attention Deficit Hyperactivity Disorder', *ADHD Attention Deficit and Hyperactivity Disorders*, 2 (2010), pp. 241–55.

2 Russell Barkley, *Attention-deficit Hyperactivity Disorder: A Handbook for Diagnosis and Treatment*, 3rd edn (New York, 2006), pp. 3–52; Wikipedia, 'History of Attention-Deficit Hyperactivity Disorder', at http://en.wikipedia.org, accessed 23 December 2010.

3 Erica D. Palmer and Stanley Finger, 'An Early Description of ADHD (Inattentive Subtype): Dr Alexander and "Mental Restlessness" (1798)', *Child Psychology and Psychiatry Review*, 6 (2001), pp. 66–73.

4 Russell Barkley, *ADHD and the Nature of Self Control* (New York, 1997); Michael Fitzgerald, 'Wolfgang Amadeus Mozart: The Allegro Composer', *Canadian Journal of Diagnosis*, 17 (2000), pp. 61–4; Paul H. Wender, *ADHD: Attention-Deficit Hyperactivity Disorder in Children and Adults* (Oxford, 2000); Michael Fitzgerald, 'Did Lord Byron Have Attention Deficit Hyperactivity Disorder?', *Journal of Medical Biography*, 9 (2001), pp. 31–3; A. Siddiqui and M. Fitzgerald, 'Did Sir Winston Churchill Have Hyperkinetic or Bipolar Affective Disorder?', *European Journal of Child and Adolescent Psychiatry*, 12 (2003), p. 219; R. Doyle, 'The History of Adult Attention-Deficit/ Hyperactivity Disorder, *Psychiatric Clinics of North America*, 27 (2004), pp. 203–14; George Capaccio, *ADD and ADHD* (Tarrytown, NY, 2008).

5 B. Raymond Hoobler, 'Some Early Symptoms Suggesting Protein Sensitization in Infancy', *American Journal of Diseases of Children*, 12 (1916), pp. 129–35; T. Wood Clarke, 'Neuro-Allergy in Childhood', *New York State Journal of Medicine*, 42 (1948), pp. 393–7.

6 W. Ray Shannon, 'Neuropathic Manifestations in Infants and Children as a Result of Anaphylactic Reaction to Foods Contained in Their Dietary', *American Journal of Disease of Children*, 24 (1922), pp. 89–94; Walter C. Alvarez, 'Puzzling "Nervous Storms" Due to Food Allergy', *Gastroenterology*, 7 (1946), pp. 241–52; Theron G. Randolph, 'Allergy as a Causative Factor of Fatigue, Irritability, and Behavior Problems of Children', *Journal of Pediatrics*, 31 (1947), pp. 560–72; T. W. Clarke, 'The Relation of Allergy to Character

Problems in Children', *Annals of Allergy*, 8 (1950), pp. 175–87.

7 Anne Applebaum, 'The ADHD-ventures of Tom Sawyer', *Slate* (9 August 2010), at www.slate.com, accessed 22 December 2010.

8 German Berrios, '"Mind in General" By Sir Alexander Crichton', *History of Psychiatry*, 17 (2006), p. 471.

9 Palmer and Finger, 'An Early Description', pp. 66–73.

10 Alexander Crichton, *An Inquiry into the Nature and Origin of Mental Derangement Comprehending a Concise System of the Physiology and Pathology of the Human Mind and a History of the Passions and Their Effects* (London, 1798), p. 254.

11 Ibid., p. 271.

12 Italics in original. Ibid., pp. 271–2.

13 Ibid., pp. 255–6.

14 Ibid., pp. 258–9.

15 Ibid., p. 267.

16 Ibid., p. 268.

17 Ibid., p. 260.

18 Ibid., p. 277.

19 Ibid., p. 278.

20 Ibid., p. 280.

21 Ibid., p. 276.

22 Ibid., pp. 271–5.

23 Ibid., p. 271.

24 Russell A. Barkley, 'Commentary on Excerpt of Crichton's Chapter, On Attention and Its Diseases', *Journal of Attention Disorders*, 12 (2008), p. 206.

25 Heinrich Hoffmann, *Struwwelpeter: Merry Stories and Funny Pictures* (New York, [1844] 1848), at www.gutenberg.org, accessed 10 January 2011.

26 Jack Zipes, *Sticks and Stones: The Troublesome Success of Children's Literature from Slovenly Peter to Harry Potter* (New York, 2002), p. 131.

27 Hoffmann, *Struwwelpeter*.

28 Margaret R. Higonnet, 'Civility Books, Child Citizens, and Uncivil Antics', *Poetics Today*, 13 (1992), p. 133.

29 Ibid.

30 Ibid., p. 134.

31 J. Thome and K. A. Jacobs, 'Attention Deficit Hyperativity Disorder

(ADHD) in a 19th Century Children's Book', *European Psychiatry*, 19 (2004), pp. 303–6.

32 Ibid., p. 305.

33 Seija Sandberg and Joanne Barton, 'Historical Development', in *Hyperactivity and Attention Disorders of Childhood*, ed. Seija Sandberg (Cambridge, 2002), pp. 1–29.

34 Thomas S. Clouston, 'Stages of Overexcitability, Hypersensitiveness and Mental Explosiveness and Their Treatment by the Bromides', *Scottish Medical and Surgical Journal*, 4 (1899), p. 483.

35 Ibid.

36 Ibid., p. 485.

37 D. A. Jackson and A. R. King, 'Gender Differences in the Effects of Oppositional Behavior on Teacher Ratings of ADHD Symptoms', *Journal of Abnormal Child Psychology*, 32 (2004), pp. 215–24.

38 Clouston, 'Stages of Overexcitability', p. 489.

39 George F. Still, 'The Goulstonian Lectures on Some Abnormal Psychical Conditions in Children', *Lancet*, 159 (1902), p. 1008.

40 One exception to this is sociologist Adam Rafalovich. See Adam Rafalovich, 'The Conceptual History of Attention-Deficit/Hyper-activity Disorder: Idiocy, Imbecility, Encephalitis, and the Child Deviant, 1877–1929', *Deviant Behavior*, 22 (2001), pp. 93–115.

41 Still, 'Goulstonian Lectures', p. 1008.

42 Ibid., p. 1009.

43 Ibid.

44 Ibid., p. 1079.

45 Mark Jackson, *The Borderland of Imbecility: Medicine, Society and the Fabrication of the Feeble Mind in Late Victorian and Edwardian England* (Manchester, 2000), pp. 1–5.

46 Ibid., 12.

47 Ibid., p. 28.

48 Eric G. L. Bywaters, 'George Frederic Still (1868–1941): His Life and Work', *Journal of Medical Biography*, 2 (1994), pp. 125–31.

49 F. T. Thorpe, 'Prefrontal Leucotomy in Treatment for Post-encephalitic Conduct Disorder', *British Medical Journal*, 1 (1946), pp. 312–14.

50 Franklin G. Ebaugh, 'Neuropsychiatric Sequelae of Acute Epidemic Encephalitis in Children', *American Journal of Diseases of Children*, 25

(1923), pp. 89–90.

51 Ibid., pp. 90–96.

52 See Jack D. Pressman, *Last Resort: Psychosurgery and the Limits of Medicine* (Cambridge, 1998).

53 Thorpe, 'Prefrontal Leucotomy', pp. 312–14.

54 Still, 'Goulstonian Lectures', pp. 1077–8.

55 Eugen Kahn and Louis Cohen, 'Organic Drivenness: A Brain-stem Syndrome and an Experience with Case Reports', *New England Journal of Medicine*, 210 (1934), pp. 748–56; Alfred A. Strauss and Heinz Werner, 'Disorders of Conceptual Thinking in the Brain-injured Child', *Journal of Nervous and Mental Disease*, 96 (1942), pp. 153–72.

56 Myerson quoted in Rick Mayes and Adam Rafalovich, 'Suffer the Restless Children: The Evolution of ADHD and Paediatric Stimulant Use, 1900–1980', *History of Psychiatry*, 18 (2007), p. 442.

57 This contrasts somewhat with sociologist Ilina Singh's suggestion that Bradley Home was 'grounded in a combination of behaviorist, psychoanalytic, and mental hygienist principles', although Bradley's 'more active biomedical interventions' are discussed. Ilina Singh, 'Bad Boys, Good Mothers, and the "Miracle" of Ritalin', *Science in Context*, 15 (2002), p. 589.

58 Anonymous, 'Images in Psychiatry: Charles Bradley, MD, 1902–1979', *American Journal of Psychiatry*, 155 (1998), p. 968; Charles Bradley, 'The Behavior of Children Receiving Benzedrine', *American Journal of Psychiatry*, 94 (1937), pp. 577–85; Charles Bradley, 'Benzedrine and Dexedrine in the Treatment of Children's Behavior Disorders', *Pediatrics*, 5 (1950), pp. 24–37.

59 Mayes and Rafalovich, 'Suffer the Restless Children', p. 443.

60 Anonymous, 'Images in Psychiatry', p. 968.

61 Rafalovich, 'Conceptual History', p. 95.

TWO: The First Hyperactive Children

1 Carol Ann Winchell, *The Hyperkinetic Child: A Bibliography of Medical, Educational, and Behavioral Studies* (Greenwood, CT, 1975).

2 David Healy, *The Antidepressant Era* (Cambridge, MA, 1997).

3 Herb Kutchins and Stuart A. Kirk also discuss the emergence of PTSD and the expansion of the DSM more generally, implicating the

role of the American Psychiatric Association. Herb Kutchins and Stuart A. Kirk, *Making Us Crazy: DSM – The Psychiatric Bible and the Creation of Mental Disorders* (New York, 1997).

4 Allan Young, *The Harmony of Illusions: The Invention of Post-traumatic Stress Disorder* (Princeton, NJ, 1995), p. 5.

5 Ibid., p. 290.

6 Michael W. Otto, Aude Henin, Dina R. Hirshfeld-Becker, Mark H. Pollack, Joseph Biederman and Jerrold F. Rosenbaum, 'Postraumatic Stress Disorder Symptoms following Media Exposure to Tragic Events: Impact of 9/11 on Children at Risk for Anxiety Disorders', *Journal of Anxiety Disorders*, 21 (2007), pp. 888–902; Allan Young, 'Who Put the Stress on Post-traumatic Stress and What Makes It Work?', seminar presented at the University of Exeter, 11 November 2008.

7 Richard Noll, *American Madness: The Rise and Fall of Dementia Praecox* (Cambridge, MA, 2011); Young, *Harmony of Illusions*.

8 David Healy, *Mania: A Short History of Bipolar Disorder* (Baltimore, MD, 2008), pp. 135–60.

9 Kay Redfield Jamison, *Touched with Fire: Manic Depressive Illness and the Artistic Temperament* (New York, 1994).

10 David Healy, 'The Latest Mania: Selling Bipolar Disorder', *PLoS Medicine*, 3 (2006), p. 0443.

11 Ibid., p. 0442.

12 Maurice W. Laufer, Eric Denhoff and Gerald Solomons, 'Hyper-kinetic Impulse Disorder in Children's Behavior Problems', *Psychosomatic Medicine*, 19 (1957), p. 41; Rick Mayes and Adam Rafalovich, 'Suffer the Restless Children: The Evolution of ADHD and Paediatric Stimulant Use, 1900–1980', *History of Psychiatry*, 18 (2007), p. 444.

13 Laufer, Denhoff and Solomons, 'Hyperkinetic Impulse Disorder', pp. 39, 43.

14 Maurice W. Laufer and Eric Denhoff, 'Hyperkinetic Behavior Syndrome in Children', *Journal of Pediatrics*, 50 (1957), pp. 463–74; Laufer, Denhoff and Solomons, 'Hyperkinetic Impulse Disorder'.

15 Laufer, Denhoff and Solomons, 'Hyperkinetic Impulse Disorder', pp. 39, 48.

16 Howard Fischer, '50 Years Ago in the *Journal of Pediatrics*: Hyper-kinetic Behavior Syndrome in Children', *Journal of Pediatrics*, 150

(2007), p. 520.

17 Laufer, Denhoff and Solomons, 'Hyperkinetic Impulse Disorder',
    p. 41.

18 Ibid., p. 45.

19 Laufer and Denhoff, 'Hyperkinetic Behavior Syndrome', p. 463.

20 Laufer, Denhoff and Solomons, 'Hyperkinetic Impulse Disorder',
    p. 44.

21 Ibid., p. 41.

22 Ibid., pp. 44–6.

23 Justin M. Call, 'Some Problems and Challenges in the Geography of
    Child Psychiatry', *Journal of the American Academy of Child Psychiatry*, 15
    (1976), p. 156.

24 Ilana Löwy, 'The Strength of Loose Concepts – Boundary Concepts,
    Federative Experimental Strategies and Disciplinary Growth: The
    Case of Immunology', *History of Science*, 30 (1992), pp. 371–3.

25 Ibid., pp. 45–8.

26 James J. McCarthy, 'SEIMCS [Special Education Instruction Materials
    Centers] and the Teacher of Children with Learning Disabilities: A
    Useful Partnership', *Exceptional Children*, 34 (1967/8), p. 627.

27 Leo Kanner, *Child Psychiatry*, 3rd edn (Springfield, IL, 1957), p. 528;
    Jules Schrager, Janet Lindy, Saul Harrison, John McDermott and Paul
    Wilson, 'The Hyperkinetic Child: An Overview of the Issues', *Journal
    of the American Academy of Child Psychiatry*, 5 (1966), p. 528.

28 Gerald Grob, *The Mad among Us: A History of the Care of America's
    Mentally Ill* (New York, 1994), p. 193.

29 Palmer Hoyt, 'What Is Ahead for Our Schools', *Grade Teacher*, 76
    (1958–9), p. 20.

30 Mark Jackson, *The Borderland of Imbecility: Medicine, Society and the
    Fabrication of the Feeble Mind in Late Victorian and Edwardian England*
    (Manchester, 2000), p. 1.

31 Ibid., p. 2.

32 Ibid., p. 12.

33 William W. Brickman, 'Educational Developments in the United
    States during 1957 and 1958', *International Review of Education*, 5
    (1959), pp. 117–18.

34 Vital Statistics of the United States, 'Live Births, Birth Rates, and
    Fertility Rates, by Race of Child: United States, 1909–80', at

www.cdc.gov, accessed 9 February 2011.

35 Irving Bernstein, *Promises Kept: John F. Kennedy's New Frontier* (New York, 1991), p. 219; Elaine Tyler May, *Homeward Bound: American Families in the Cold War Era*, 2nd edn (New York, [1988] 1999), pp. 76, 120–21; Doug Owram, *Born at the Right Time: A History of the Baby-boom Generation* (Toronto, 1996), pp. 6, 116.

36 Paul L. Gardner, 'Guidance: An Orientation for the Classroom Teacher', *Clearing House*, 36 (1961/2), p. 38.

37 Betty Barton and Katharine D. Pringle, 'Today's Children and Youth: I. As Viewed from the States', *Children*, 7 (1960), p. 54.

38 Laufer, Denhoff and Solomons, 'Hyperkinetic Impulse Disorder', 46.

39 Steven Mintz and Susan Kellogg, *Domestic Revolutions: A Social History of Family Life* (New York, 1988), pp. 184–7.

40 Franklin G. Ebaugh, 'Comment: The Case of the Confused Parent', *American Journal of Psychiatry*, 116 (1960), p. 1136.

41 Gerald L. Gutek, *Education in the United States: An Historical Perspective* (Englewood Cliffs, NJ, 1986), pp. 279–80.

42 Steven A. Modée, 'Post Sputnik Panic', *English Journal*, 69 (1980), p. 56, reproduced with permission of the National Council of Teachers of English.

43 Barbara Ehrenreich and Deirdre English, *For Her Own Good: 150 Years of the Experts' Advice to Women* (Garden City, NY, 1979), p. 232. Ironically, Dennis's father, Henry, was an aerospace engineer.

44 Alice V. Keliher, 'I Wonder as I Wander', *Grade Teacher*, 76 (1958–9), p. 143.

45 Harold G. Shane, 'Elementary Schools during the Fabulous Fifties', *The Education Digest*, 26 (1961), p. 19; Toni Taylor, 'Editorial: Take a Good Look This Year', *Grade Teacher*, 76 (1958–9), p. 5.

46 Erik Erikson, 'Youth and the Life Cycle', *Children*, 7 (1960), p. 49.

47 Diane Ravitch, *The Troubled Crusade: American Education, 1945–1980* (New York, 1983), pp. 43–6.

48 Time Magazine, 'Progressive Education in the 1940s', at www.youtube.com, accessed 9 February 2011.

49 Stanley E. Ballinger, 'John Dewey: Man Ahead of His Times', *The Education Digest*, 25 (1959–60), pp. 9–11.

50 Ibid.

51 Ibid.

52 Ehrenreich and English, *For Her Own Good*, pp. 226–39.

53 Hoyt, 'What Is Ahead', p. 20.

54 Hyman G. Rickover, *American Education – A National Failure: The Problem of Our Schools and What We Can Learn from England* (New York, 1963), p. 32.

55 Capitals in original. Asa S. Knowles, 'For the Space Age: Education as an Instrument of National Policy', *Phi Delta Kappa*, 39 (1958), p. 306.

56 Lloyd Berkner quoted in Rickover, *American Education*, p. 57.

57 Arthur S. Trace, *What Ivan Knows That Johnny Doesn't* (New York, 1961), p. 3.

58 Anonymous, 'Education: What Ivan Reads', *Time* (17 November 1961), at www.time.com, accessed 11 February, 2011.

59 Rickover, *American Education*, p. 71.

60 James Bryant Conant, *The American High School Today: A First Report to Interested Citizens* (New York, 1959), pp. 45–50, 55–6.

61 Barbara Barksdale Clowse, *Brainpower for the Cold War: The Sputnik Crisis and the National Defense Education Act of 1958* (Westport, CT, 1981); Wayne J. Urban, *More Than Science and Sputnik: The National Defense Education Act of 1958* (Tuscaloosa, AL, 2010).

62 Arthur S. Flemming, 'The Philosophy and Objectives of the National Defense Education Act', *Annals of the American Academy of Political and Social Science*, 327 (1960), p. 132.

63 Ibid., p. 134.

64 Gerard de Groot, *Dark Side of the Moon: The Magnificent Madness of the American Lunar Quest* (New York, 2006).

65 Anthony Davids and Jack Sidmond, 'A Pilot Study – Impulsivity, Time Orientation, and Delayed Gratification in Future Scientists and in Underachieving High School Students', *Exceptional Children*, 29 (1962/3), p. 170.

66 Ibid., p. 174.

67 Phyllis O. Edwards, 'Discipline and the Elementary School', *Grade Teacher*, 74 (1956–7), p. 129.

68 Norma E. Cutts, 'Troublesome or Troubled', *Grade Teacher*, 76 (1958–9), p. 56; Alice V. Keliher, 'You, the Psychologist and the Child', *Grade Teacher*, 74 (1956–7), p. 143; Sol Cohen, 'The Mental Hygiene Movement, the Development of Personality and the School:

The Medicalization of American Education', *History of Education Quarterly*, 23 (1983), p. 35.

69 Gregory Rochlin, 'Discussion of David E. Reiser's "Observations of Delinquent Behavior in Very Young Children"', *Journal of the American Academy of Child Psychiatry*, 2 (1963), p. 66.

70 Keliher, 'You, the Psychologist and the Child', p. 143.

71 Katherine Reeves, 'Each in His Own Good Time', *Grade Teacher*, 74 (1956–7), p.8.

72 Reeves, 'Each in His Own', p. 117.

73 Peter Conrad and Deborah Potter, 'From Hyperactive Children to ADHD Adults: Observations on the Expansion of Medical Categories', *Social Problems*, 47 (2000); Sigmund Gundle, 'Discussion of Masterson, Tucker and Berk's "Psychopathology in Adolescence, IV: Clinical and Dynamic Characteristics"', *American Journal of Psychiatry*, 120 (1963/4), p. 365; James F. Masterson, Jr, 'The Symptomatic Adolescent Five Years Later: He Didn't Grow out of It', *American Journal of Psychiatry*, 123 (1966/7), pp. 1338, 1345; James F. Masterson, Jr, Kenneth Tucker and Gloria Berk, 'Psychopathology in Adolescence, IV: Clinical and Dynamic Characteristics', *American Journal of Psychiatry*, 120 (1963/4), p. 363.

74 Masterson, Jr, 'The Symptomatic Adolescent', pp. 1338–44.

75 Barton and Pringle, 'Today's Children and Youth', p. 55; Alice V. Keliher, 'You and the Psychological Experts', *Grade Teacher*, 74 (1956–7), p. 113; Edward A. Richards, 'Today's Children and Youth: II. As Seen by National Organizations', *Children*, 7 (1960), p. 60.

76 These advertisements began in the 1956–7 volume of *Grade Teacher*.

77 R. H. Eckelberry, 'Editorial Comment: A Year of the Space Age', *Educational Research Bulletin*, 37 (1958), p. 222.

78 Viscount Hailsham quoted in Alice K. Smith, 'Eggheads of the World, Unite!', *Bulletin of the Atomic Scientists*, 14 (1958), p. 151.

79 Daniel Schreiber, 'The Dropout and the Delinquent: Promising Practices Gleaned from a Year of Study', *Phi Delta Kappa*, 44 (1963), p. 217.

80 Stafford L. Warren, 'Implementation of the President's Program on Mental Retardation', *American Journal of Psychiatry*, 121 (1964/5), pp. 550–51.

81 Lyndon B. Johnson quoted in Daniel Schreiber, 'The Low-down on

Dropouts', in PTA *Guide to What's Happening in Education*, ed. Eva H. Grant (New York, 1965), p. 245.

82 Jane D. McLeod and Karen Kaiser, 'Childhood Emotional and Behavioral Problems and Educational Attainment', *American Sociological Review*, 69 (2004); Kathleen G. Nadeau, 'Career Choices and Workplace Challenges for Individuals with ADHD', *Journal of Clinical Psychology*, 61 (2005); Lester Tarnapol, 'Author's Comment', *Exceptional Children*, 36 (1969/70), p. 368.

83 Schreiber, 'The Low-down', p. 246; Daniel W. Snepp, 'Can We Salvage the Drop-outs?', *Clearing House*, 31 (1956/7), p. 49; Claudia Goldin, 'America's Graduation from High School: The Evolution and Spread of Secondary Schooling in the Twentieth Century', *Journal of Economic History*, 58 (1998), pp. 345–7.

84 Schreiber, 'The Low-down', p. 246–7.

85 US Department of Veterans Affairs, 'GI Bill History', at www.gibill.va.gov, accessed 14 February 2011.

86 Rickover, *American Education*, pp. 50–51.

87 James Bryant Conant, *Slums and Suburbs* (New York, 1961), p. 145.

88 Ibid.

89 Eli Ginzberg and Marcia Freedman, 'Problems of Educational and Vocational Development in Adolescence' in *The Psychopathology of Adolescence*, ed. Joseph Zubin and Alfred M. Freedman (New York, 1970), pp. 79–81.

90 Marsh F. Beall, 'Disenchanted Students', *Science*, 175 (1972), p. 123.

91 Dorothy Barclay, 'A Turn for the Wiser', *Pediatrics*, 23 (1959), p. 760.

92 K. Minde, D. Lewin, Gabrielle Weiss, H. Lavigueur, Virginia Douglas and Elizabeth Sykes, 'The Hyperactive Child in Elementary School: A 5 Year, Controlled, Followup', *Exceptional Children*, 38 (1971/2), pp. 219, 221.

93 Ibid., p. 221.

94 Conant, *Slums and Suburbs*, pp. 2–3.

95 Lloyd M. Dunn, 'Special Education for the Mildly Retarded – Is Much of It Justifiable?' *Exceptional Children*, 35 (1968/9), p. 20.

96 Ernest Siegel, 'Learning Disabilities: Substance or Shadow', *Exceptional Children*, 34 (1967/8), p. 436.

97 Howard S. Adelman, 'The Not So Specific Learning Disability Population', *Exceptional Children*, 37 (1970/71), p. 530.

98 Thomas C. Lovitt, 'Assessment of Children with Learning Disabilities', *Exceptional Children*, 34 (1967/8), p. 237.

99 James Bryant Conant, 'Recommendations for the Junior-High School', *The Education Digest*, 26 (1961), p. 7.

100 Conant, *American High School Today*, pp. 44–5.

101 Sabrina E. B. Schuck and Francis M. Crinella, 'Why Children with ADHD Do Not Have Low IQs', *Journal of Learning Disabilities*, 38 (2005), pp. 262–80.

102 S. Alexander Rippa, *Education in a Free Society: An American History*, 7th edn (New York, 1992), pp. 262–3.

103 I. N. Berlin, 'Mental Health Consultation in Schools as a Means of Communicating Mental Health Principles', *Journal of the American Academy of Child Psychiatry*, 1 (1962), pp. 674–5; P. J. Doyle, 'The Organic Hyperkinetic Syndrome', *Journal of School Health*, 32 (1962), pp. 299, 304; Paul L. Gardner, 'Guidance: An Orientation for the Classroom Teacher', *Clearing House*, 36 (1961/2); Eva H. Grant, 'Forward', in PTA *Guide to What's Happening in Education*, ed. Eva H. Grant (New York, 1965), p. iii; T. P. Millar, 'Schools Should Not Be Community Health Centers', *American Journal of Psychiatry*, 125 (1968/9), p. 119; Emily Mumford, 'Teacher Response to School Mental Health Problems', *American Journal of Psychiatry*, 125 (1968/9), pp. 76–8.

104 Rema Lapouse and Mary A. Monk, 'An Epidemiologic Study of Behavior Characteristics in Children', *American Journal of Public Health*, 48 (1958), p. 1134; Keliher, 'You, the Psychologist and the Child', p. 143; William W. Wattenberg, 'Mental Health and Illness', *The Education Digest*, 26 (1961), p. 11.

105 Lovitt, 'Assessment of Children', p. 234.

106 Eric Denhoff, 'To Medicate – to Debate – or to Validate', *Journal of Learning Disabilities*, 4 (1971), p. 469.

107 Ibid.

108 Doyle, 'The Organic Hyperkinetic Syndrome', p. 304; Barbara K. Keogh, 'Hyperactivity and Learning Disorders: Review and Speculation', *Exceptional Children*, 38 (1971/2), p. 101; H. G. Wadsworth, 'A Motivational Approach Towards Remediation of Learning Disabled Boys', *Exceptional Children*, 38 (1971/2), pp. 32–4.

109 John Peterson, 'The Researcher and the Underachiever: Never the

Twain Shall Meet', *Phi Delta Kappa*, 44 (1963), p. 381.

110 Peter Schrag and Diane Divoky, *The Myth of the Hyperactive Child: And Other Means of Child Control* (New York, [1975] 1982), pp. 111–15. See, for example, the increase in advertisements during the 1970s for hyperactivity drugs such as Ritalin and Cylert in journals such as the *American Journal of Psychiatry*.

111 J. Michael Coleman and Earl E. Davis, 'Learning Disabilities: Ten Years Later', *Peabody Journal of Education*, 53 (1976), p. 180.

112 Association of American Universities, 'A National Defense Education Act for the 21st Century Renewing Our Commitment to U.S. Students, Science, Scholarship, and Security' (2006), at www.aau.edu, accessed 11 February 2011; Association of American Universities, 'National Defense Education and Innovation Initiative – Meeting America's Economic and Security Initiatives in the 21st Century' (2006), at www.aau.edu, accessed 11 February 2011.

113 George S. Counts, 'The Real Challenge of Soviet Education', *The Education Digest*, 25 (1959–60), p. 8.

114 Allan V. Horwitz, *Creating Mental Illness* (Chicago, IL, 2003), pp. 18–20.

115 Italics in original. Harry Hendrick, *Child Welfare: Historical Dimensions, Contemporary Debate* (Bristol, 2003), p. 253.

THREE: Debating Hyperactivity

1 American Psychiatric Association (APA), *Diagnostic and Statistical Manual of Mental Disorders*, 2nd edn (Washington, DC, 1968), p. 50.

2 Dominick Calobrisi, 'Classification of Children's Mental Disorders', *American Journal of Psychiatry*, 125 (1968/9), p. 1458.

3 Ibid., pp. 31–2.

4 Ibid.

5 Ibid., pp. 49–51.

6 Richard L. Jenkins, 'More on Diagnostic Nomenclature', *American Journal of Psychiatry*, 125 (1968/9), p. 1603.

7 Charles E. Rosenberg, *Explaining Epidemics and Other Studies in the History of Medicine* (Cambridge, 1992), pp. 245–56. See also Gerald N. Grob, *From Asylum to Community: Mental Health Policy in Modern America* (Princeton, NJ, 1991), pp. 51, 279.

8 Christopher J. Wardle, 'Review of a Neuropsychiatric Study in

Childhood', *British Journal of Psychiatry*, 119 (1971), p. 565.

9 Roy Porter and Mark S. Micale, 'Introduction: Reflection on Psychiatry and Its Histories', in *Discovering the History of Psychiatry*, ed. Roy Porter and Mark S. Micale (Oxford, 1994), pp. 5–6.

10 See Jack D. Pressman, *Last Resort: Psychosurgery and the Limits of Medicine* (Cambridge, 1998).

11 See Thomas Szasz, 'Psychiatry, Ethics and Criminal Law', *Columbia Law Review*, 58 (1958), pp. 183–98; R. D. Laing, *The Divided Self: An Existential Study in Sanity and Madness* (Harmondsworth, 1960); Erving Goffman, *Asylums: Essays on the Social Situation of Mental Patients and Other Inmates* (Garden City, NY, 1962); Ken Kesey, *One Flew over the Cuckoo's Nest* (New York, 1962); Michel Foucault, *Madness and Civilization: A History of Insanity in the Age of Reason*, trans. Richard Howard (New York, 1965).

12 Howard P. Rome, 'Psychiatry Viewed from the Outside: The Challenge of the Next Ten Years', *American Journal of Psychiatry*, 123 (1967/8), p. 519.

13 Gerald N. Grob, 'Government and Mental Health Policy: A Structural Approach', *The Millbank Quarterly*, 72 (1994), p. 481.

14 Nathan G. Hale, *The Rise and Crisis of Psychoanalysis in the United States* (Oxford, 1995), p. 381.

15 Robert H. Felix, 'State Planning for Participation in the National Mental Health Act', *Public Health Reports*, 62 (1947), pp. 1183, 1191.

16 Gerald N. Grob, 'Creation of the National Institutes of Mental Health', *Public Health Reports*, 111 (1996), pp. 378–80.

17 Grob, 'Government and Mental Health Policy', p. 484.

18 Ibid., p. 485.

19 Reginald S. Lourie, 'The Joint Commission on the Mental Health of Children', *American Journal of Psychiatry*, 122 (1965/6), p. 1280.

20 Charles Hersch, 'The Clinician and the Joint Commission Report: A Dialogue', *Journal of the American Academy of Child Psychiatry*, 10 (1971), p. 407.

21 John F. Kennedy, 'Message from the President of the United States Relative to Mental Illness and Mental Retardation', *American Journal of Psychiatry*, 120 (1963/4), p. 729.

22 C. H. Hardin Branch, 'Presidential Address: Preparedness for Progress', *American Journal of Psychiatry*, 120 (1963/4), p. 2.

23 Ibid.

24 Council of the APA, 'A Tribute to John Fitzgerald Kennedy', *American Journal of Psychiatry*, 120 (1963/4), unnumbered addendum between pp. 728 and 729.

25 Pressman, *Last Resort*, pp. 355–6.

26 Grob, *From Asylum to Community*, p. 100; Hale, *Rise and Crisis*; Edward Shorter, *A History of Psychiatry* (New York, 1997); John J. Leveille, 'Jurisdictional Competition and the Psychoanalytic Dominance of American Psychiatry', *Journal of Historical Sociology*, 15 (2002), p. 252.

27 Leveille, 'Jurisdictional Competition', pp. 252–3.

28 Eveoleen N. Rexford, 'A Developmental Concept of the Problem of Acting Out', *Journal of the American Academy of Child Psychiatry*, 2 (1963), pp. 6–21; Charles A. Malone, 'Some Observations on Children of Disorganized Families and Problems of Acting Out', *Journal of the American Academy of Child Psychiatry*, 2 (1963), pp. 22–49; David E. Reiser, 'Observations of Delinquent Behavior in Very Young Children', *Journal of the American Academy of Child Psychiatry*, 2 (1963), pp. 50–71.

29 Albert J. Solnit, 'Who Deserves Child Psychiatry? A Study in Priorities', *Journal of the American Academy of Child Psychiatry*, 5 (1966), p. 3.

30 Mark A. Stewart, 'Correspondence: Dynamic Orientation', *American Journal of Psychiatry*, 117 (1960), p. 85.

31 L. Borje Lofgren, 'A Comment on "Swedish Psychiatry"', *American Journal of Psychiatry*, 116 (1959), pp. 83–4.

32 Rexford, 'A Developmental Concept', pp. 9–10; Reiser, 'Observations of Delinquent Behavior', pp. 50, 53, 67; Jules Schrager, Janet Lindy, Saul Harrison, John McDermott and Paul Wilson, 'The Hyperkinetic Child: An Overview of the Issues', *Journal of the American Academy of Child Psychiatry*, 5 (1966), p. 529; D. S. Leventhal, 'The Significance of Ego Psychology for the Concept of Minimal Brain Dysfunction in Children', *Journal of the American Academy of Child Psychiatry*, 7 (1968), pp. 242–51; C. M. Heinicke and L. H. Strassman, 'Toward More Effective Research on Child Psychotherapy', *Journal of the American Academy of Child Psychiatry*, 14 (1975), pp. 561–88.

33 George A. Rogers, 'Methylphenidate Interviews in Psychotherapy', *American Journal of Psychiatry*, 117 (1960/1), p. 549; W. Smith, 'Trifluoperazine in Children and Adolescents with Marked Behavior Problems', *American Journal of Psychiatry*, 121 (1964/5), p. 703.

34 J. Weinreb and R. M. Counts, 'Impulsivity in Adolescents and Its Therapeutic Management', *Archives of General Psychiatry*, 2 (1960), pp. 549–50.

35 Alexander Thomas, Herbert Birch, Stella Chess and Lillian C. Robbins, 'Individuality in Responses of Children to Similar Environmental Situations', *American Journal of Psychiatry*, 116 (1960), p. 798; Rexford, 'A Developmental Concept', pp. 10–11; Reiser, 'Observations of Delinquent Behavior', p. 53.

36 Rexford, 'A Developmental Concept', p. 11; Adelaide M. Johnson and S. A. Szurek, 'The Genesis of Antisocial Acting Out in Children and Adults', in *Learning and Its Disorder: Clinical Approaches to the Problems of Childhood*, ed. Irving N. Berlin and S. A. Szurek (Palo Alto, CA, 1965), p. 136; Esther S. Battle and Beth Lacey, 'A Context for Hyperactivity in Children over Time', *Child Development*, 43 (1972), pp. 757, 772.

37 Kathleen W. Jones, *Taming the Troublesome Child: American Families, Child Guidance and the Limits of Psychiatric Authority* (Cambridge, MA, 1999), p. 210.

38 Heather Munro Prescott, *A Doctor of Their Own: The History of Adolescent Medicine* (Cambridge, MA, 1998), p. 108.

39 E. Kahn, 'Is Psychotherapy Science?', *American Journal of Psychiatry*, 117 (1960/1), p. 755; Henry A. Davidson, 'The Image of the Psychiatrist', *American Journal of Psychiatry*, 121 (1964/5), pp. 329–34; Robert H. Felix, 'The Image of the Psychiatrist: Past, Present and Future', *American Journal of Psychiatry*, 121 (1964/5), p. 319; Leon Eisenberg, 'Discussion of Dr. Solnit's Paper "Who Deserves Child Psychiatry? A Study in Priorities"', *Journal of the American Academy of Child Psychiatry*, 5 (1966), p. 20; Judd Marmor, 'The Current Status of Psychoanalysis in American Psychiatry', *American Journal of Psychiatry*, 125 (1968/9), p. 679.

40 John S. Werry, 'The Use of Psychotropic Drugs in Children', *Journal of the American Academy of Child Psychiatry*, 16 (1977), p. 463.

41 Jonathan Michel Metzl, *Prozac on the Couch: Prescribing Gender in the Era of Wonder Drugs* (Durham, NC, 2003), p. 35.

42 Solnit, 'Who Deserves Child Psychiatry', p. 3.

43 Eisenberg, 'Discussion', pp. 20–21.

44 E. A Grootenboer, 'The Relation of Housing to Behavior Disorder', *American Journal of Psychiatry*, 119 (1962/3), p. 471; Malone, 'Some

Observations', pp. 22–3; Stella Chess, Alexander Thomas and Herbert G. Birch, 'Behavior Problems Revisited: Findings of an Anteroperspective Study', *Journal of the American Academy of Child Psychiatry*, 6 (1967), p. 330; John P. Spiegel, 'Social Change and Unrest: The Responsibility of the Psychiatrist', *American Journal of Psychiatry*, 125 (1967/8), pp. 1580–81.

45 Anonymous quoted in Henry A. Davidson, 'Comment: The Reversible Superego', *American Journal of Psychiatry*, 120 (1963/4), p. 192.

46 Eisenberg, 'Discussion', p. 23.

47 Hersch, 'The Clinician and the Joint Commission', p. 411.

48 S. A. Cermak, F. Stein and C. Abelson, 'Hyperactive Children and an Activity Group Therapy Model', *American Journal of Occupational Therapy*, 27 (1973), pp. 311–15.

49 Harold B. Levy, 'Amphetamines in Hyperkinetic Children', *Journal of the American Medical Association*, 216 (1971), p. 1865.

50 Ibid.

51 Eveoleen N. Rexford, 'Child Psychiatry and Child Analysis in the United States', *Journal of the American Academy of Child Psychiatry*, 1 (1962), p. 381.

52 Paulina F. Kernberg, 'The Problem of Organicity in the Child: Notes on Some Diagnostic Techniques in the Evaluation of Children', *Journal of the American Academy of Child Psychiatry*, 8 (1969), p. 537.

53 One exception, which might help to explain why play therapy was not used more often, is described in N. Carrey, 'Interview with Dr. Gabrielle "Gaby" Weiss', *Journal of the Canadian Academy of Child and Adolescent Psychiatry*, 18 (2004), p. 341.

54 Anna Freud, *Normality and Pathology in Childhood* (New York, 1965); Irwin Jay Knopf, *Childhood Psychopathology: A Developmental Approach* (Englewood Cliffs, NJ, 1979), pp. 165–6.

55 Leon Eisenberg, Anita Gilbert, Leon Cytryn and Peter A. Molling, 'The Effectiveness of Psychotherapy Alone and in Conjunction with Perphenazine or Placebo in the Treatment of Neurotic and Hyperactive Children', *American Journal of Psychiatry*, 116 (1960), p. 1092; Sidney Berman, 'Techniques of Treatment of a Form of Juvenile Delinquency, the Antisocial Character Disorder', *Journal of the American Academy of Child Psychiatry*, 3 (1964), p. 24; Edmund F. Kal, 'Organic Versus Functional Diagnoses', *American Journal of Psychiatry*,

125 (1969), p. 1128; Judith Rapoport, Alice Abramson, Duane Alexander and Ira Lott, 'Playroom Observations of Hyperactive Children on Medication', *Journal of the American Academy of Child Psychiatry*, 10 (1971), p. 531.

56　Kennedy, 'Message from the President', pp. 729–37.

57　Will Bradbury, 'An Agony of Learning', *Life* (October 1972); Irving Berstein, *Promises Kept: John F. Kennedy's New Frontier* (New York, 1991), p. 243.

58　Robert E. L. Faris and H. Warren Dunham, *Mental Disorders in Urban Areas* (Chicago, IL, 1939); August B. Hollingshead and Frederick C. Redlich, *Social Class and Mental Illness: A Community Study* (New York, 1958); Alexander Leighton, *My Name is Legion: Foundations for a Theory of Man in Relation to Culture* (New York, 1959); Leo Srole, Thomas S. Langner, Stanley T. Michael, Marvin K. Opler and Thomas A. C. Rennie, *Mental Health in the Metropolis: The Midtown Manhattan Study* (New York, 1962).

59　Spiegel, 'Social Change', pp. 1581–2; Leonard Duhl, 'Dr Duhl Replies', *American Journal of Psychiatry*, 123 (1966/7), pp. 701–11; Henry W. Brosin, 'Response to the Presidential Address', *American Journal of Psychiatry*, 124 (1967/8), p. 7.

60　APA, 'Position Statement on Crisis in Child Mental Health: Challenge for the 1970s, Final Report of the Joint Commission on the Mental Health of Children', *American Journal of Psychiatry*, 125 (1968/9), pp. 1197–1203.

61　Kennedy, 'Message from the President', p. 737.

62　Branch, 'Presidential Address', p. 10; Jack R. Ewalt, 'Presidential Address', *American Journal of Psychiatry*, 121 (1964/5), p. 980; Daniel Blain, 'Presidential Address: Novalescence', *American Journal of Psychiatry*, 122 (1965/6), p. 4; Henry W. Brosin, 'Presidential Address: Adaptation to the Unknown', *American Journal of Psychiatry*, 125 (1968/9), p. 7; Raymond S. Waggoner, Sr, 'Presidential Address: Cultural Dissonance and Psychiatry', *American Journal of Psychiatry*, 127 (1970/1), p. 1.

63　Anonymous, 'Editorial Statement', *Social Psychiatry*, 1 (1966), p. 1.

64　Sir David Henderson quoted in Joshua Bierer, 'Introduction to the Second Volume', *International Journal of Social Psychiatry*, 2 (1956), p. 8.

65　B. Lieber, 'Letter to the Editor', *International Journal of Social Psychiatry*,

2 (1956), pp. 235–7.

66 Michael Harrington, *The Other America* (New York, 1962).

67 Hans Selye, *The Stress of Life* (London, 1957).

68 Malone, 'Some Observations', pp. 22–3; Grootenboer, 'Relation of Housing', p. 471; George E. Gardner, 'Aggression and Violence – The Enemies of Precision Learning in Children', *American Journal of Psychiatry*, 128 (1971/2), p. 446.

69 Anonymous, 'Millions of Children Need Psychiatric Aid', JAMA, 209 (1969), p. 356.

70 Stella Chess, Alexander Thomas, Michael Rutter and Herbert G. Birch, 'Interaction of Temperament and Environment in the Production of Behavior Disturbances in Children', *American Journal of Psychiatry*, 120 (1963/4), p. 147.

71 Irving N. Berlin, 'The Atomic Age, the Nonlearning Child, the Parent', in *Learning and Its Disorders: Clinical Approaches to Problems of Childhood*, ed. Irving N. Berlin and S. A. Szurek (Palo Alto, CA, 1965), p. 84; Chess, Thomas and Birch, 'Behavior Problems Revisited', p. 330.

72 E. A. Goldstein and Leon Eisenberg, 'Child Psychiatry, Mental Deficiency', *American Journal of Psychiatry*, 121 (1964/5), pp. 655–6.

73 Eisenberg, 'Discussion', p. 23; Leon Eisenberg quoted in Jules Schrager, Janet Lindy, Saul Harrison, John McDermott and Wilson, 'The Hyperkinetic Child Syndrome: An Overview of the Issues', *Journal of the American Academy of Child Psychiatry*, 6 (1966), p. 530. See also Leon Eisenberg, 'Foreword', in *Formative Years: Children's Health in the United States, 1880–2000*, ed. Alexandra Minna Stern and Howard Markel (Ann Arbor, MI, 2002), pp. viii–xvi.

74 Irving Philips, Herbert C. Modlin, Irving N. Berlin, Leon Eisenberg, Howard P. Rome and Raymond W. Waggoner, 'The Psychiatrist, the APA, and Social Issues: A Symposium', *American Journal of Psychiatry*, 128 (1971/2), p. 684.

75 Berlin, 'Atomic Age', pp. 65–6.

76 Eleanor Pavenstedt, 'Introduction to the Symposium on Research on Infancy and Early Childhood', *Journal of the American Academy of Child Psychiatry*, 1 (1962), pp. 5–10; Eleanor Pavenstedt, 'Psychiatric Services for Underprivileged Children', *International Psychiatry Clinics*, 8 (1971), pp. 101–41.

77 Malone, 'Some Observations', pp. 22–3.

78 Lourie, 'Joint Commission', p. 1280.

79 APA, 'Position Statement', pp. 1197–8.

80 Joseph D. Noshpitz, 'Toward a National Policy for Children', *Journal of the American Academy of Child Psychiatry*, 13 (1974), p. 390.

81 David L. Bazelon, 'The Problem Child – Whose Problem?', *Journal of the American Academy of Child Psychiatry*, 13 (1974), p. 199.

82 Brosin, 'Response', pp. 7–8.

83 Brosin, 'Presidential Address', p. 5.

84 John W. Gardner quoted in Brosin, 'Presidential Address', p. 7.

85 Solnit, 'Who Deserves Child Psychiatry?', p. 7.

86 Ibid., p. 2.

87 Leo H. Bartemeier, 'The Future of Psychiatry: The Report on the Joint Commission on Mental Illness and Health', *American Journal of Psychiatry*, 16 (1959/60), p. 978.

88 Oscar B. Markey, 'Bridges or Fences?', *Journal of the American Academy of Child Psychiatry*, 2 (1963), p. 375; Edward J. A. Nuffield, 'Child Psychiatry Limited: A Conservative Viewpoint', *Journal of the American Academy of Child Psychiatry*, 7 (1968), pp. 217–21; Robert M. Eisendrath, 'A Lack of Zip and a Sense of Gold', *American Journal of Psychiatry*, 123 (1967/8), p. 708.

89 C. Keith Conners, 'Symptom Patterns in Hyperkinetic, Neurotic, and Normal Children', *Child Development*, 41 (1970), pp. 677–8.

90 John I. Langdell, 'Phenylketonuria: Some Effects of Body Chemistry on Learning', *Journal of the American Academy of Child Psychiatry*, 6 (1967), p. 166.

91 Rapoport et al., 'Playroom Observations', p. 524.

92 John S. Werry, 'An Overview of Pediatric Psychopharmacology', *Journal of the American Academy of Child Psychiatry*, 21 (1982), p. 3.

93 C. Keith Conners and Leon Eisenberg, 'The Effects of Methylphenidate on Symptomology and Learning in Disturbed Children', *American Journal of Psychiatry*, 120 (1963), p. 458.

94 Don Mahler, 'Review of the Film: *The Hyperactive Child*', *Exceptional Children*, 38 (1971/2), p. 161; Schrag and Divoky, *The Myth of the Hyperactive Child*, pp. 80–84.

95 Dorothea M. Ross and Sheila A. Ross, *Hyperactivity: Research, Theory, and Action* (New York, 1976), p. 99.

96 David Herzberg, *Happy Pills in America: From Miltown to Prozac* (Baltimore, MD, 2009), p. 27

97 Andrea Tone, *The Age of Anxiety: A History of America's Turbulent Affair with Tranquilizers* (New York, 2009); Nicolas Rasmussen, *On Speed: The Many Lives of Amphetamine* (New York, 2008).

98 JAMA, 209 (1969), pp. 609–10.

99 Leonard Cammer, 'Treatment Methods and Fashions in Treatment', *American Journal of Psychiatry*, 118 (1961/2), p. 448.

100 Ilina Singh, 'Bad Boys, Good Mothers, and the "Miracle" of Ritalin', *Science in Context*, 15 (2002), p. 593.

101 Eric Denhoff quoted in Robert Reinhold, 'Drugs That Help to Control the Unruly Child', *New York Times* (5 July 1970), p. 96.

102 Anonymous, 'Drugs Seem to Help Hyperactive Children', JAMA, 214 (1970), p. 2262; Larry B. Silver, 'The Playroom Diagnostic Evaluation of Children with Neurologically Based Learning Disabilities', *Journal of the American Academy of Child Psychiatry*, 15 (1976), p. 253; Leighton Y. Huey, Mark Zetin, David S. Jankowsky and Lewis L. Judd, 'Adult Minimal Brain Dysfunction and Schizophrenia', *American Journal of Psychiatry*, 134 (1977), pp. 1563–5; Werry, 'Use of Psychotropic Drugs', p. 453.

103 Leon Tec, 'An Additional Observation on Methylphenidate in Hyperactive Children', *American Journal of Psychiatry*, 127 (1970/1), p. 1424.

104 Maurice Laufer in Anonymous, 'Drugs Seem to Help Hyperactive Children', JAMA, 214 (1970), p. 2262; B. D. Garfinkel, C. D. Webster and L. Sloman, 'Methylphenidate and Caffeine in the Treatment of Children with Minimal Brain Dysfunction', *American Journal of Psychiatry*, 132 (1975), p. 723; A. R. Lucas and M. Weiss, 'Methylphenidate Hallucinosis', JAMA, 217 (1971) , pp. 1079–81.

105 Joaquim Puig-Antich, Laurence L. Greenhill, Jon Sassin, Edward J. Sachar, 'Growth Hormone, Prolactin and Cortisol Responses and Growth Patterns in Hyperkinetic Children Treated with Dextro-Amphetamine', *Journal of the American Academy of Child Psychiatry*, 17 (1976), p. 457.

106 Joseph O. Cole, 'Psychopharmacology: The Picture Is Not Entirely Rosy', *American Journal of Psychiatry*, 127 (1971), pp. 224–5.

107 Robert L. Spitzer and Dennis P. Cantwell, 'The DSM-III Classification of Psychiatric Disorders of Infancy, Childhood, and

Adolescence', *Journal of the American Academy of Child Psychiatry*, 18 (1979), pp. 356–70.

108 Werry, 'Overview', pp. 3, 8.

109 Michael Rutter and David Shaffer, 'DSM-III: A Step Forward or Back in Terms of the Classification of Child Psychiatric Disorders', *Journal of the American Academy of Child Psychiatry*, 18 (1979), pp. 371–94.

110 Spitzer and Cantwell, 'DSM-III', p. 363.

111 Felix, 'Image of the Psychiatrist', pp. 318–22.

112 Allan V. Horwitz, 'Pharmaceuticals and the Medicalization of Social Life', in *The Risks of Prescription Drugs*, ed. Donald W. Light (New York, 2010), p. 94.

113 Nick Clegg quoted in 'Nick Clegg on Mental Health Investment', BBC News, 2 February 2011, at www.bbc.co.uk, accessed 7 March 2011.

FOUR: Ritalin: Magic Bullet or Black Magic?

1 Rock Brynner and Trent Stephens, *Dark Remedy: The Impact of Thalidomide and Its Revival as a Vital Medicine* (Cambridge, MA, 2001), pp. 122–61.

2 See James Mills, *Cannabis Britannica: Empire, Trade and Prohibition, 1800–1928* (Oxford, 2005); Virginia Berridge, *Opium and the People* (London, 1999).

3 James Mills, 'Cannabis in the Commons; Colonial Networks, Missionary Politics and the Origins of the Indian Hemp Drugs Commission 1893–4', *Journal of Colonialism and Colonial History*, 6 (2005).

4 Erika Dyck, *Psychedelic Psychiatry: LSD from Clinic to Campus* (Baltimore, MD, 2008), p. 53.

5 Ibid., p. 73.

6 Ibid., pp. 103–7.

7 Nicolas Rasmussen, *On Speed: The Many Lives of Amphetamine* (New York, 2008), p. 219.

8 Richard L. Myers, *The 100 Most Important Chemical Compounds* (Westport, CT, 2007), p. 178.

9 Ibid.; C. Stier, 'The Use of Ritalin, a Central Nervous System Stimulant, in Depressive States and for the Support of Electric Shock

Therapy', *Therapie der Gegenwart*, 94 (1955), pp. 92–5; George A. Rogers, 'Methylphenidate Interviews in Psychotherapy', *American Journal of Psychiatry*, 117 (1960/1), pp. 549–50.

10 Rasmussen, *On Speed*, pp. 27–35, 149–52.

11 Ilina Singh, 'Not Just Naughty: Fifty Years of Stimulant Drug Advertising', in *Medicating Modern America*, ed. Andrea Tone and Elizabeth Siegel Watkins (New York, 2007), pp. 134–5.

12 Nathan William Moon, 'The Amphetamine Years: A Study of the Medical Applications and Extramedical Consumption of Psycho-stimulant Drugs in the Postwar United States, 1945–1980', PhD thesis, Georgia Tech University, 2009, p. 56.

13 Moon, 'Amphetamine Years', pp. 150–52.

14 David Healy, *The Antidepressant Era* (Cambridge, MA, 1997), pp. 43–5.

15 Peter Schrag and Diane Divoky, *The Myth of the Hyperactive Child: And Other Means of Child Control* (New York, [1975] 1981), p. 84; Walter Sneader, *Drug Discovery: A History* (Chichester, 2005), pp. 432–45.

16 Anonymous, 'New Drug Rouses Mental Patients', *The Science News-Letter*, 68 (1955), p. 184; Anonymous, 'Drugs Check Oldsters Behavior Problems', *The Science News-Letter*, 68 (1955), p. 373; Anonymous, 'Drugs Help Oldsters', *The Science News-Letter*, 69 (1956), p. 68; Chauncy D. Leake, 'Newer Stimulant Drugs', *American Journal of Nursing*, 58 (1958), pp. 966–8.

17 Nancy Tomes, 'The Great American Medicine Show Revisited', *Bulletin of the History of Medicine*, 79 (2005), p. 635.

18 Ibid.

19 Moon, 'Amphetamine Years', p. 131.

20 Ibid., p. 56.

21 Christopher Windham, 'Ritalin Shows Promise in Treating Lethargy, Depression in Elderly', *Wall Street Journal* (17 July 2003), at www.aegis.org, accessed 15 March 2011; K. Ritchie, S. Artero, F. Portet, A. Brickman, J. Muraskin, E. Beanino, M. L. Ancelin and L. Carrière, 'Caffeine, Cognitive Functioning, and White Matter Lesions in the Elderly: Establishing Causality from Epidemiological Evidence', *Journal of Alzheimers Disease*, 20 (2010), pp. s161–6.

22 J. Leslie LeHew quoted in Moon, 'Amphetamine Years', p. 75.

23 Edward Shorter, *Before Prozac: The Troubled History of Mood Disorders in Psychiatry* (Oxford, 2009), pp. 39–41; Moon, 'Amphetamine Years',

pp. 57–9, 63–8, 79–83.

24 Anonymous, 'Images in Psychiatry: Charles Bradley, MD, 1902–1979', *American Journal of Psychiatry*, 155 (1998), p. 968.

25 C. Keith Conners and Leon Eisenberg, 'The Effects of Methylphenidate on Symptomology and Learning in Disturbed Children', *American Journal of Psychiatry*, 120 (1963/4), p. 458.

26 Peter Conrad, 'The Discovery of Hyperkinesis: Notes on the Medicalization of Deviant Behavior', *Social Problems*, 23 (1975), p. 16.

27 Frederic T. Zimmerman and Bessie B. Burgemeister, 'Action of Methyl-Phenidylacetate (Ritalin) and Resperine in Behavior Disorders of Children and Adults', *American Journal of Psychiatry*, 115 (1958/9), p. 325.

28 J. G. Millichap, 'The Paradoxical Effects of CNS Stimulants on Hyperkinetic Behavior', *International Journal of Neurology*, 10 (1975), pp. 241–51; M. J. Millard and L. J. Sandish, 'The Paradoxical Effect of Central Nervous System Stimulants on Hyperactivity: A Paradox Unexplained by the Rate-dependent Effect', *Journal of Nervous and Mental Disorders*, 170 (1982), pp. 499–501; C. E. Drouin, M. Page and B. D. Waterhouse, 'Methylphenidate Enhances Noradrenergic Transmission and Suppresses Mid- and Long-Latency Sensory Responses in the Primary Somatosensory Cortex of Awake Rats', *Journal of Neurophysiology*, 96 (2006), pp. 622–32.

29 George Lytton and Mauricio Knobel, 'Diagnosis and Treatment of Behavior Disorders in Children', *Diseases of the Nervous System*, 20 (1959), pp. 334–40.

30 Leon Eisenberg, Anita Gilbert, Leon Cytryn, Peter A. Molling, 'The Effectiveness of Psychotherapy Alone and in Conjunction with Perphenazine or Placebo in the Treatment of Neurotic and Hyper-kinetic Children', *American Journal of Psychiatry*, 116 (1959), pp. 1088–93.

31 Ibid., p. 1092.

32 Conners and Eisenberg, 'Effects of Methylphenidate', pp. 458–64.

33 Ibid., p. 458.

34 Leon Eisenberg, Roy Lachman, Peter A. Molling, Arthur Lockner, James D. Mizelle and C. Keith Conners, 'A Psychopharmacologic Experiment in a Training School for Delinquent Boys', *American Journal of Orthopsychiatry*, 33 (1963), pp. 431–47.

35 Conners and Eisenberg, 'Effects of Methylphenidate', p. 460.

36 Ibid., p. 461.

37 Zimmerman and Burgemeister, 'Action of Methyl-Phenidylacetate', p. 323; Joel Zrull, Jack C. Westman, Bettie Arthur and Dale L. Rice, 'A Comparison of Diazepam, D-Amphetamine, and Placebo in the Treatment of Hyperkinetic Syndrome in Children', *American Journal of Psychiatry*, 121 (1964/5), pp. 388–9; Gabrielle Weiss, Klaus Minde, Virginia Douglas, John Werry and Donald Sykes, 'Comparison of the Effects of Chlorpromazine, Dextroamphetamine and Methylphenidate on the Behaviour and Intellectual Functioning of Hyperactive Children', *Canadian Medical Association Journal*, 104 (1971), pp. 20–25.

38 Conners and Eisenberg, 'Effects of Methylphenidate', p. 462. Conners's caution foreshadows his role in the controversy over the Feingold diet and hyperactivity a decade later. Conners was one of the few researchers involved in the debates who vacillated regarding Feingold's hypothesis that food additives triggered hyperactivity. His opinion on the matter shifted back and forth numerous times, testifying not to his indecision, but his recognition of the highly complex nature of Feingold's hypothesis and how to test it (see chapter Five for more details). It should also be remembered that Eisenberg was one of the few biological psychiatrists who heartily supported the theory behind and action endorsed by social psychiatry.

39 Joel P. Zrull, 'Discussion', *American Journal of Psychiatry*, 120 (1963/4), pp. 463–4.

40 Robert Reinhold, 'Drugs That Help to Control the Unruly Child', *New York Times* (5 July 1970), p. 96.

41 Ibid.

42 Ibid.

43 Robert Reinhold, 'Rx for Child's Learning Malady', *New York Times* (3 July 1970), p. 27.

44 Ibid.

45 Ibid.

46 It is interesting that the two articles just cited, both written by Robert Reinhold, were published days after another article in the *New York Times*, written by another journalist, reporting that there would be a government study into fears that Ritalin was being over-prescribed.

47 Richard D. Young quoted in Robert Reinhold, 'Learning Parley

Divided on Drugs', *New York Times* (6 February 1968), p. 40.

48 Sidney J. Adler quoted in Reinhold, 'Learning Parley', p. 40.

49 Ibid.

50 Constance Holden, 'Amphetamines: Tighter Controls on the Horizon', *Science*, 194 (1976), pp. 1027–8; Rasmussen, *On Speed*, pp. 182–221.

51 Lester Grinspoon and Peter Hedblom, *Speed Culture: Amphetamine Use and Abuse in America* (Cambridge, MA, 1975), p. 11.

52 Harold M. Schmeck, Jr, 'Tighter Control Asked on 2 Drugs', *New York Times* (17 July 1971), p. 8.

53 Ibid.

54 Rasmussen, *On Speed*, p. 219.

55 Reinhold, 'Rx', p. 27.

56 Schrag and Divoky, *Myth of the Hyperactive Child*, p. 84; Leighton Y. Huey, Mark Zetin, David S. Janowsky and Lewis L. Judd, 'Adult Minimal Brain Dysfunction and Schizophrenia: A Case Report', *American Journal of Psychiatry*, 134 (1977), p. 1563; Stella Chess and Susan G. Gordon, 'Psychosocial Development and Human Variance', *Review of Research in Education*, 11 (1984), p. 35.

57 Robert M. Veatch, 'Drugs and Competing Drug Ethics', *Hastings Center Studies*, 2 (1974), p. 72.

58 Grinspoon and Hedblom, *Speed Culture*, p. 228.

59 Nat Hentoff, 'Drug-Pushing in the Schools: The Professionals (1)', *Village Voice* (25 May 1972), p. 21.

60 Ibid.

61 Schrag and Divoky, *Myth of the Hyperactive Child*, p. 84.

62 Leon Oettinger quoted in Schrag and Divoky, *Myth of the Hyperactive Child*, p. 85.

63 Ibid., p. 112.

64 Ibid., pp. 84–5, 111–16.

65 Ibid., pp. 111–12, 115–16.

66 Will Bradbury, 'An Agony of Learning', *Life* (14 October 1973).

67 Robert L. Sprague and Kenneth D. Gadow, 'The Role of the Teacher in Drug Treatment', *School Review*, 85 (1976), p. 121.

68 Weiss et al., 'Comparison of the Effects', p. 24.

69 Ibid.

70 Ibid., p. 20.

71 L. Oettinger, Jr and L. V. Majovski, 'Methylphenidate: A Review', *Southern Medical Journal*, 69 (1976), pp. 161–3.

72 J. O. Cole, 'Hyperkinetic Children: The Use of Stimulant Drugs Evaluated', *American Journal of Orthopsychiatry*, 45 (1975), pp. 28–37; M. Schleifer, G. Weiss, N. Cohen, M. Elman, E. Kruger, 'Hyperactivity in Preschoolers and the Effect of Methylphenidate', *American Journal of Orthopsychiatry*, 45 (1975), pp. 38–50.

73 Patricia O. Quinn and Judith L. Rapoport, 'One-Year Follow-up of Hyperactive Boys Treated with Imipramine or Methylphenidate', *American Journal of Psychiatry*, 132 (1975), pp. 241–5; Fay Shafto and Stephen Sulzbacher, 'Comparing Treatment Tactics with a Hyperactive Preschool Child: Stimulant Medication and Programmed Teacher Intervention', *Journal of Applied Behavior Analysis*, 10 (1977), pp. 13–20.

74 Leon Tec, 'An Additional Observation on Methylphenidate in Hyperactive Children', *American Journal of Psychiatry*, 127 (1970/1), p. 1424; Roger D. Freeman, 'Minimal Brain Dysfunction, Hyperactivity, and Learning Disorders: Epidemic or Episode?', *School Review*, 85 (1976), pp. 9–10; John S. Werry, 'The Use of Psychotropic Drugs in Children', *Journal of the American Academy of Child Psychiatry*, 16 (1977), p. 451.

75 Robert C. Schnackenberg, 'Caffeine as a Substitute for Schedule II Stimulants in Hyperkinetic Children', *American Journal of Psychiatry*, 130 (1973), pp. 796–8.

76 David Pineda, Alfredo Ardila, Monica Rosselli, Beatriz E. Arias, Gloria C. Henao, Luisa F. Gomez, Sylvia E. Mejia and Martha L. Miranda, 'Prevalence of Attention-Deficit/Hyperactivity Disorder Symptoms in 4- to 17-year-old Children in the General Population', *Journal of Abnormal Child Psychology*, 27 (1999), pp. 455–62.

77 Barry D. Garfinkel, Christopher D. Webster and Leon Sloman, 'Methylphenidate and Caffeine in the Treatment of Children with Minimal Brain Dysfunction', *American Journal of Psychiatry*, 132 (1975), pp. 723–8.

78 Robert D. Huestis, L. Eugene Arnold and Donald J. Smeltzer, 'Caffeine Versus Methylphenidate and d-Amphetamine in Minimal Brain Dysfunction: A Double-blind Comparison', *American Journal of Psychiatry*, 132 (1975), pp. 868–70; Philip Firestone, Jean Davey, John

T. Goodman and Susan Peters, 'The Effects of Caffeine and Methylphenidate on Hyperactive Children', *Journal of the American Academy of Child Psychiatry*, 17 (1978), pp. 445–56.

79 Richard A. Johnson, James B. Kenney and John B. Davis, 'Developing School Policy for Use of Stimulant Drugs for Hyperactive Children', *The School Review*, 85 (1976), p. 82.

80 Robert Maynard, 'Omaha Pupils Given "Behavior" Drugs', *Washington Post* (29 June 1970), p. A1; United States Congressional House Government and Operations Committee, 'Federal Involvement in the Use of Behavior Modification Drugs on Grammar School Children in the Right to Privacy Inquiry', 91st Congress, 2nd Session (Washington, DC, 1970).

81 Johnson, Kenney and Davis, 'Developing School Policy', pp. 91–2.

82 Ibid., p. 78.

83 H. Lennard, L. Epstein, A. Bernstein and D. Ransom, 'Hazards Implicit in Prescribing Psychoactive Drugs', *Science*, 169 (1970), pp. 438–41.

84 Mark Stewart quoted in Anonymous, 'Classroom Pushers', *Time* (26 February 1973), at www.time.com, accessed 23 March 2011.

85 Freeman, 'Minimal Brain Dysfunction', p. 11.

86 Klaus K. Minde, 'The Hyperactive Child', *Canadian Medical Association Journal*, 112 (1975), p. 130.

87 Ibid.

88 Fred F. Glancy, Jr, quoted in Diane Divoky, 'Learning-disability "Epidemic"', *New York Times* (15 January 1975), p. 61.

89 John Hurst quoted in Anonymous, 'Classroom Pushers'.

90 T. Paramenter quoted in Johnson, Kenney and Davis, 'Developing School Policy', pp. 80–81.

91 Anonymous, 'Classroom Pushers'.

92 Ibid.

93 Rasmussen, *On Speed*, pp. 233–4.

94 Ibid.

95 Minde, 'Hyperactive Child', p. 130.

96 Stanley Krippner, Robert Silverman, Michael Cavallo and Michael Healy, 'Stimulant Drugs and Hyperkinesis: A Question of Diagnosis', *Literacy Research and Instruction*, 13 (1974), p. 219.

97 Lawrence Diller, 'The Run on Ritalin: Attention Deficit Disorder and

Stimulant Treatment in the 1990s', *The Hastings Center Report*, 26 (1996), p. 12.

98 Maurice Laufer quoted in Reinhold, 'Drugs that Help Control the Unruly Child', p. 96.

99 Daniel M. Martin quoted in Anonymous, 'Those Mean Little Kids', *Time* (18 October 1968), at www.time.com, accessed 29 March 2011.

100 James Swanson quoted in Jonathan Leo, 'American Preschoolers on Ritalin', *Society* (January/February 2002), p. 53.

101 Sidney Adler quoted in Anonymous, 'Drugs for Learning', *Time* (10 August 1970), at www.time.com, accessed 29 March 2011.

102 Maurice Laufer quoted in Anonymous, 'Drugs for Learning'.

103 Adam Rafalovich, 'Disciplining Domesticity: Framing the ADHD Parent and Child', *Sociological Quarterly*, 42 (2001), p. 379.

104 Anonymous, 'Mean Little Kids'.

105 Ilina Singh, 'Bad Boys, Good Mothers, and the "Miracle" of Ritalin', *Science in Context*, 15 (2002), pp. 577–603.

106 Christopher McAllister, 'The (Re)Legitimization of State Violence in Britain and the USA', in *(Re)Constructing Cultures of Violence and Peace*, ed. Richard Jackson (Amsterdam, 2004), p. 46.

107 Ilina Singh and Kelly Kelleher, 'Neuroenhancement in Young People: Proposal for Research, Policy, and Clinical Management', *AJOB Neuroscience*, 1 (2010), p. 3.

108 Ibid., p. 9.

109 Steve Salvatore, 'Group Issues Guidelines for Monitoring Ritalin in Children', CNN International Edition online (9 November 1998), at www.edition.cnn.com, accessed 20 March 2011.

110 Fred A. Baughman, Jr, *The ADHD Fraud: How Psychiatry Makes 'Patients' out of Normal Children* (Victoria, BC, 2006), p.1.

111 Lawrence Smith, 'Death from Ritalin: The Truth behind ADHD', at www.ritalindeath.com, accessed 4 April 2011.

112 Thomas E. Wilens, Jefferson B. Prince, Thomas J. Spencer and Joseph Biederman, 'Stimulants and Sudden Death: What Is a Physician to Do?', *Pediatrics*, 118 (2006), p. 1215.

113 Steven E. Nissen, 'ADHD Drugs and Cardiovascular Risk', *New England Journal of Medicine*, 354 (2006), pp. 1147–8.

114 Leslie Iverson, *Speed, Ecstasy, Ritalin: The Science of Amphetamines* (Oxford, [2006] 2008), p. 64.

115 Matthew Knight, 'Stimulant Drug Therapy for Attention-Deficit Disorder (with or without Hyperactivity) and Sudden Cardiac Death', *Pediatrics*, 119 (2007), pp. 154–5.

116 Wilens et al., 'Stimulants and Sudden Death', p. 1215.

117 Lydia Furman, 'Stimulants and Sudden Death: What Is the Real Risk?' *Pediatrics*, 119 (2007), p. 409.

118 Leo, 'American Preschoolers on Ritalin', p. 55.

119 Rasmussen, *On Speed*, p. 259.

FIVE: Alternative Approaches

1 Cleo Jeppson quoted in Elaine Jarvik, 'The Calming of the Hyperactive', *Utah Holiday* (May 1978), p. 48.

2 Jarvik, 'Calming of the Hyperactive', p. 50.

3 William McLennand, 'Hyperactive Children', *American Psychologist*, 35 (1980) pp. 392–3.

4 L. Eugene Arnold, 'Alternative Treatments for Adults with Attention-Deficit Hyperactivity Disorder (ADHD)', *Annals of the New York Academy of Sciences*, 931 (2001), pp. 310–41.

5 Francis Hare, *The Food Factor in Disease* (London, 1905); B. Raymond Hoobler, 'Some Early Symptoms Suggesting Protein Sensitization in Infancy', *American Journal of Diseases of Children*, 12 (1916), pp. 129–33; W. Ray Shannon, 'Neuropathic Manifestations in Infants and Children as a Result of Anaphylactic Reaction to Foods Contained in Their Dietary', *American Journal of Disease of Children*, 24 (1922), pp. 89–94; Arthur C. Coca, *Familial Nonreaginic Food-allergy* (Springfield, IL, 1943); Albert H. Rowe, *Clinical Allergy Due to Foods, Inhalants, Contactants, Fungi, Bacteria and Other Causes* (London, 1937); Theron G. Randolph, 'Allergy as a Causative Factor of Fatigue, Irritability and Behavior Problems of Children', *Journal of Pediatrics*, 31 (1947), pp. 560–72; H. M. Davison, 'Cerebral Allergy', *Southern Medical Journal*, 42 (1949), pp. 712–16. Other allergists, particularly those influenced by psychoanalysis, believed that the relationship flowed in the other direction. Allergies were a psychosomatic phenomenon triggered by emotional disturbance. Carla Keirns, 'Better Than Nature: The Changing Treatment of Asthma and Hay Fever in the United States, 1910–1945', *Studies in History and*

Philosophy of Biological and Biomedical Sciences, 34 (2003), pp. 511–31; Mark Jackson, '"Allergy Con Amore": Psychosomatic Medicine and the "Asthmogenic Home" in the Mid-twentieth Century', in Health and the Modern Home, ed. Mark Jackson (New York, 2007), pp. 153–74.

6 Shannon, 'Neuropathic Manifestations', p. 91.

7 T. Wood Clarke, 'The Relation of Allergy to Character Problems in Children: A Survey', Annals of Allergy, 8 (1950), pp. 175–87.

8 Ibid., p. 178.

9 Frederic Speer, 'The Allergic Tension-Fatigue Syndrome in Children', International Archives of Allergy and Applied Immunology, 12 (1958), pp. 207–14.

10 William G. Crook, Walton W. Harrison and Stanley E. Crawford, 'Allergy – The Unanswered Challenge in Pediatric Research, Education and Practice', Pediatrics, 21 (1958), pp. 649–54.

11 Theron G. Randolph, 'Clinical Ecology as It Affects the Psychiatric Patient', International Journal of Social Psychiatry, 12 (1966), p. 251.

12 M. A. Stewart, 'Hyperactive Children', Scientific American, 222 (1970), p. 94; Oliver J. David, 'Association between Lower Level Lead Concentrations and Hyperactivity in Children', Environmental Health Perspectives, 7 (1974), pp. 17–25.

13 R. R. Byers quoted in David, 'Lower Lead Concentrations', pp. 18–19.

14 David, 'Lower Lead Concentrations'.

15 E. K. Silbergeld and A. M. Goldberg, 'Hyperactivity: A Lead-induced Behavior Disorder', Environmental Health Perspectives, 7 (1974), pp. 227–32.

16 David, 'Lower Lead Concentrations', p. 24.

17 C. J. Bullpitt, 'Lead and Hyperactivity', Lancet (25 November 1972), p. 1144.

18 D. Krehbiel, G. A. Davis, L. M. LeRoy and R. E. Bowman, 'Absence of Hyperactivity in Lead-exposed Developing Rats', Environmental Health Perspectives, 18 (1976), pp. 147–57.

19 J. T. Nigg, M. Nikolas, G. Mark Knottnerus, K. Cavanagh and K. Friderici, 'Confirmation and Extension of Association of Blood Level Lead with Attention-Deficit/Hyperactivity Disorder (ADHD) and ADHD Symptom Domains and Population-typical Exposure Levels', Journal of Child Psychology and Psychiatry, 51 (2010), pp. 58–65; Paul A. Eubig, Andréa Aguiar and Susan L. Schantz, 'Lead and PCBs as Risk

Factors for Attention Deficit/Hyperactivity Disorder', *Environmental Health Perspectives*, 118 (2010), pp. 1654–67; Anonymous, 'Poisoning the Mind', *The Economist* (4 February 2010).

20 Nachum Vaisman, Nehemia Kaysar, Yahalomit Zaruk-Adasha, Dori Pelled, Gérard Brichon, Georges Zwingelstein and Jacques Bodennec, 'Correlation between Changes in Blood Fatty Acid Composition and Visual Sustained Attention Performance in Children with Inattention: Effect of Dietary n–3 Fatty Acids Containing Phospholipids', *American Journal of Clinical Nutrition*, 87 (2008), pp. 1070–80; M. Arns, S. de Ridder, M. Breteler and A. Coenen, 'Efficacy of Neurofeedback Treatment in ADHD: The Effects on Inattention, Impulsivity and Hyperactivity: A Meta-analysis', *Clinical EEG and Neuroscience*, 40 (2009), pp. 180–89; J. Rucklidge, M. Taylor and K. Whitehead, 'Effect of Micronutrients on Behavior and Mood in Adults with ADHD: Evidence from an 8-Week Open Label Trial with Natural Extension', *Journal of Attention Disorders*, 15 (2011), pp. 79–91.

21 For more on the history of the Feingold hypothesis, see: Matthew Smith, *An Alternative History of Hyperactivity: Food Additives and the Feingold Diet* (New Brunswick, NJ, 2011).

22 Benjamin F. Feingold, *Why Your Child Is Hyperactive* (New York, 1974), pp. 1–3.

23 Feingold, *Why Your Child Is Hyperactive*, p. 11

24 Ibid., p. 17.

25 Feingold's theory was also reported in less reputable publications, such as the *National Enquirer* and *Penthouse*.

26 Morton Mintz, 'Study Links Food Additives to Hyperactive Children', *Washington Post* (29 October 1973), pp. A1, A9; United States Congress, 'Food Additives and Hyperactivity in Children', USA Congressional Record 119 (30 October 1973), pp. S1936–19742.

27 Ben F. Feingold, *Introduction to Clinical Allergy* (Springfield, IL, 1973). Feingold's list of publications on topics unrelated to hyperactivity is too long to be listed here, but included publications in *California Medicine*, *JAMA*, *Experimental Parasitology*, *Proceedings of the Society for Experimental Biology and Medicine*, *Psychosomatic Medicine* and *Annals of Allergy*.

28 Feingold would later publish his hyperactivity theory in less

prestigious publications, such as the *Delaware Medical Journal* and *Ecology of Disease*. Ben F. Feingold, 'A View from the Other Side [A Speech to the Newspaper Food Editors and Writers Association]', (Milwaukee, WI, 8 June 1977), at www.feingold.org, accessed 4 March 2011.

29 Ben F. Feingold quoted in C. Keith Conners, *Food Additives and Hyperactive Children* (New York, 1980), p. 12.

30 John S. Werry, 'Food Additives and Hyperactivity', *Medical Journal of Australia*, 2 (1976), p. 282.

31 Harvey Levenstein, *Paradox of Plenty: A Social History of Eating in Modern America* (Oxford, 1993), p. 112.

32 NACHFA, *Report to the Nutrition Foundation* (New York, 1975).

33 NACHFA, *Final Report to the Nutrition Foundation* (New York, 1980); American Council on Science and Health, *Food Additives and Hyperactivity* (Summit, NJ, 1984); David Rosner and Gerald Markowitz, 'Industry Challenges to the Principle of Prevention in Public Health: The Precautionary Principle in Historical Perspective', *Public Health Reports*, 117 (2002), pp. 508–9.

34 Esther H. Wender, 'Food Additives and Hyperkinesis', *American Journal of Diseases of Children*, 131 (1977) pp. 1204–6. Such concerns were rebuffed in subsequent studies which calculated exactly how much vitamin C was consumed by children on the diet. Joanna Dwyer, Patricia H. Harper, Charles H. Goyette and C. Keith Conners, 'Nutrient Intakes of Children on the Hyperkinesis Diet', *Journal of the American Dietetic Association*, 73 (1980), pp. 515–20.

35 Feingold, *Why Your Child Is Hyperactive*, pp. 36–7.

36 National Institutes of Health, 'Defined Diets and Childhood Hyperactivity', NIH Consensus Statement Online, 4 (13–15 January 1982), at www.consensus.nih.gov, accessed 7 April 2011.

37 C. M. Carter, M. Urbanowicz, R. Hemsley, L. Mantilla, S. Strobel, P. J. Graham and E. Taylor, 'Effects of a Few Food Diet in Attention Deficit Disorder', *Archives of Disease in Childhood*, 69 (1993), p. 568.

38 NACHFA, *Final Report*, p. 10.

39 Bernard Rimland, 'The Feingold Diet: An Assessment of the Reviews by Mattes, by Kavale and Forness and Others', *Journal of Learning Disabilities*, 16 (1983), p. 331.

40 Terry L. Rose, 'The Functional Relationship between Artificial Food

Colors and Hyperactivity', *Journal of Applied Behavior Analysis*, 11 (1978), p. 441; James W. Swanson and Marcel Kinsbourne, 'Food Dyes Impair Performance of Hyperactive Children on a Laboratory Learning Test', *Science*, 207 (1980), pp. 1485–7.

41 NACHFA, Final Report, p. 10.

42 T. J. Sobotka, 'Estimates of Average, 90th Percentile and Maximum Daily Intakes of FD & C Artificial Food Colors in One Day's Diets among Two Age Groups of Children', *Food and Drug Administration Memorandum*, July 1976.

43 NACHFA, Final Report, p. 11.

44 Anonymous, 'Feingold's Regimen for Hyperkinesis', *Lancet*, 2 (1979), p. 617.

45 J. Preston Harley, Roberta S. Ray, Lawrence Tomasi, Peter L. Eichman, Charles G. Matthews, Raymond Chun, Charles S. Cleeland and Edward Traisman, 'Hyperkinesis and Food Additives: Testing the Feingold Hypothesis', *Pediatrics*, 61 (1978), p. 825.

46 Ben F. Feingold, 'Hyperkinesis and Learning Disabilities Linked to the Ingestion of Artificial Food Colors and Flavors', Speech to the American Academy of Pediatrics, New York Hilton Hotel, 8 November 1977, at www.feingold.org, accessed 28 January 2009; J. Ivan Williams and Douglas M. Cram, 'Diet in the Management of Hyper-kinesis: A Review of the Tests of Feingold's Hypotheses', *Canadian Psychiatric Association Journal*, 23 (1978), pp. 245–6; Bernard Weiss, 'Food Additives as a Source of Behavioral Disturbance in Children', *Neurotoxicology*, 7 (1986), p. 200.

47 Conners, *Food Additives and Hyperactive Children*, p. 39.

48 Mortimer D. Gross, Ruth A. Tofanelli, Sharyl M. Butzirus and Earl W. Snodgrass, 'The Effects of Diets Rich in and Free from Additives on the Behaviour of Children with Hyperkinetic and Learning Disorder', *Journal of the American Academy of Child and Adolescent Psychiatry*, 26 (1987), pp. 54–5.

49 Harley et al., Hyperkinesis and Learning Disabilities', p. 821; Feingold, 'Hyperkinesis and Learning Disabilities'.

50 J. A. Mattes and R. Gittelman, 'Effects of Artificial Food Colorings in Children with Hyperactive Symptoms', *Archives of General Psychiatry*, 38 (1981), p. 717.

51 C. Keith Conners, *Feeding the Brain: How Foods Affect Children* (New

York, 1989), p. 12.

52 Williams and Cram, 'Diet in the Management of Hyperkinesis', p. 243.

53 Bonnie J. Kaplan, Jane McNicol, Richard A. Conte, H. K. Moghadam, 'Dietary Replacement in Preschool-aged Hyperactive Boys', *Pediatrics*, 83 (1989), p. 7.

54 Ibid., p. 53.

55 Rimland, 'The Feingold Diet', p. 331.

56 Werry, 'Food Additives', p. 282.

57 Ibid.

58 William G. Crook, 'Adverse Reactions to Food Can Cause Hyperkinesis', *American Journal of Diseases of Childhood*, 132 (1978), pp. 819–20.

59 Feingold, *Why Your Child Is Hyperactive*, p. 160.

60 Ibid.

61 Benjamin F. Feingold, 'The Role of Diet in Behaviour', *Ecology of Disease*, 1 (1982), pp. 154–5.

62 For more on Feingold families, see Smith, *Alternative History of Hyperactivity*, chapter Eight.

63 Jeffrey A. Mattes, 'The Feingold Diet: A Current Reappraisal', *Journal of Learning Disabilities*, 16 (1983), p. 319.

64 B. Bateman, J. O. Warner, E. Hutchinson, T. Dean, P. Rowlandson, C. Grant, J. Grundy, C. Fitzgerald and J. Stephenson, 'The Effects of a Double-blind, Placebo Controlled, Artificial Food Colourings and Benzoate Preservative Challenge on Hyperactivity in a General Population Sample of Preschool Children', *Archives of Disease in Childhood*, 89 (2004), pp. 506–11.

65 Donna McCann, Angelina Barrett, Alison Cooper, Debbie Crumpler, Lindy Dalen, Kate Grimshaw, Elizabeth Kitchin, Kris Lok, Lucy Porteous, Emily Prince, Edmund Sonuga-Barke, John O. Warner and Jim Stevenson, 'Food Additives and Hyperactive Behaviour in 3-year-old and 8/9-year-old Children in the Community: A Randomised, Double-Blinded, Placebo-Controlled Trial', *Lancet*, 370 (2007), p. 1566.

66 Ibid.

67 FSA, 'FSA Advice to Parents on Food Colours and Hyperactivity', at www.food.gov.uk, accessed 14 April 2011; EFSA, 'EFSA Publishes Safety Assessments of Three Food Colours' (21 April 2010), at www.efsa.europa.eu, accessed 14 April 2011.

68 Alison Schonwald, 'ADHD and Food Additives Revisited', AAP Grand Rounds, 19 (2008), p. 17.

69 Steven Reinberg, 'FDA Panel Delays Action on Dyes Used in Foods' (31 March 2011), http://health.msn.com, accessed 14 April 2011.

SIX: Hyperactive Around the World

1 ADHD World Federation, at www.adhd-federation.org, accessed 22 November 2011.

2 Guilherme Polanczck, Maurício Silva de Lima, Bernardo Lessa Horta, Joseph Biederman and Luis Augusto Rohde, 'The Worldwide Prevalence of ADHD: A Systematic and Metaregression Analysis', American Journal of Psychiatry, 164 (2007), pp. 942–8.

3 Terrie E. Moffit and Maria Melchior, 'Why Does the Worldwide Prevalence of Childhood Attention Deficit Hyperactivity Disorder Matter?', American Journal of Psychiatry, 164 (2007), pp. 856.

4 Polanczck et al., 'Worldwide Prevalence', p. 947.

5 Steven V. Faraone, Joseph Sergeant, Christopher Gillberg and Joseph Biederman, 'The Worldwide Prevalence of ADHD: Is It an American Condition?', World Psychiatry, 2 (2003), p. 104.

6 Other researchers have done similar reviews of the epidemiological literature, but have only focused on the 1990s, which similarly skews the epidemiology of hyperactivity in the long term. Faraone et al., 'Worldwide Prevalence'.

7 Horacio Fabrega, Jr, 'Cultural and Historical Foundations of Psychiatric Diagnosis', in Culture and Psychiatric Diagnosis: A DSM-IV Perspective, ed. Juan E. Mezzich, Arthur Kleinman, Horacio Fabrega, Jr, and Delores L. Parron (Washington, DC, 1996), pp. 3–12.

8 Dana Birksted-Breen, Sarah Flanders and Alain Gibealt, eds, Reading French Psychoanalysis (London, 2009).

9 Adam Feinstein, A History of Autism: Conversations with the Pioneers (London, 2010), p. 6.

10 CDC, 'Increasing Prevalence of Parent-Reported Attention-Deficit/Hyperactivity Disorder among Children – United States, 2003 and 2007', Morbidity and Mortality Weekly Report, 59 (2010), pp. 1439–43, at www.cdc.gov, accessed 20 April 2011.

11 Dominique P. Béhague, 'Psychiatry and Politics in Pelotas, Brazil:

The Equivocal Quality of Conduct Disorder and Related Diagnoses',
Medical Anthropological Quarterly, 23 (2009), pp. 455–82.

12 See Erika Dyck and Christopher Fletcher, eds, *Locating Health: Historical
and Anthropological Investigations of Place and Health* (London, 2010).

13 M. Roy Schwartz, 'Globalization and Medical Education', *Medical
Teacher*, 23 (2001), pp. 533–4.

14 Ethan Watters, *Crazy Like Us: The Globalization of the Western Mind*
(New York, 2011). Watters' book is also published as *Crazy Like Us:
The Globalization of the American Psyche*.

15 Sami Timimi and Begum Maitra, 'ADHD and Globalization', in
Rethinking ADHD: From Brain to Culture, ed. Sami Timimi and Jonathan
Leo (Basingstoke, 2009), pp. 203–4.

16 Ibid., p. 204.

17 Ibid., p. 209.

18 Pierre Elliot Trudeau, 'Speech to the Press Club', 25 March 1969, at
http://archives.cbc.ca, accessed 21 April 2011.

19 Ed Kromer, 'Sleeping with the Elephant', *The McGill Reporter* (21
November 2002), at www.mcgill.ca, accessed 21 April 2011; CDC,
'Uninsured Americans: Newly Released Health Insurance Statistics',
at www.cdc.gov, accessed 21 April 2011.

20 Stuart Laidlaw, 'Public Health Care Scores Big as MDs Study
Privatization' (12 August 2009), at www.healthzone.ca, accessed
21 April 2011.

21 Abraham Flexner, *Medical Education in the United States and Canada*
(New York, 1910).

22 Patrick Sullivan, 'Privatization If Necessary, Not Necessarily
Privatization: CMA' (19 August 2005), at www.cma.ca, accessed
21 April 2011.

23 Sidney Katz, '"Speed" for Unruly Pupils Questioned', *Toronto Star*
(25 March 1971); Anonymous, 'Accidents in the Home Threaten the
Pre-Schooler', *Toronto Star* (22 July 1971).

24 J. Mackay, 'The Psychiatric Problems of the Teenager', *Canadian
Family Physician*, 14 (1968), pp. 21–6.

25 P. Susan Stephenson, 'Drugs in Child Psychiatry', *Canadian Family
Physician*, 15 (1969), p. 32.

26 The team's long list of hyperactivity-related publications began with
J. S. Werry, Gabrielle Weiss and Virginia Douglas, 'Studies on the

Hyperactive Child – I. Some Preliminary Findings', *Canadian Psychiatric Association Journal*, 9 (1964), pp. 120–30.

27 Gabrielle Weiss quoted in N. Carrey, 'Interview with Dr Gabrielle "Gaby" Weiss', *Journal of the Canadian Academy of Child and Adolescent Psychiatry*, 18 (2004), p. 341.

28 Oddly, Weiss's reflections about the effectiveness of Chlorpromazine differ from the findings she and her team published in other articles, which state that the drug did reduce the hyperactivity in most children studied. J. S. Werry, Gabrielle Weiss, Virginia Douglas and Judith Martin, 'Studies on the Hyperactive Child – III: The Effects of Chlorpromazine upon Behavior and Learning Ability', *Journal of the American Academy of Child Psychiatry*, 5 (1966), pp. 292–312.

29 Gabrielle Weiss, Elena Kruger, Ursel Danielson and Meryl Elman, 'Effect of Long-term Treatment of Hyperactive Children with Methylphenidate' *Canadian Medical Association Journal*, 112 (1975), pp. 159–65; L. Hechtman, G. Weiss, J. Finkelstein, A. Werner and R. Benn, 'Hyperactives as Young Adults: Preliminary Report', *Canadian Medical Association Journal*, 115 (1976), pp. 625–30; Lily Hechtman, Gabrielle Weiss, 'Long-term Outcome of Hyperactive Children', *American Journal of Orthopsychiatry*, 53 (1983), pp. 532–41.

30 Lily Hechtman, Gabrielle Weiss and Kay Metrakos, 'Hyperactive Individuals as Young Adults: Current and Longitudinal Electro-encephalographic Evaluation and Its Relation to Outcome', *Canadian Medical Association Journal*, 118 (1978), p. 919; G. Weiss, L. Hechtman, T. Perlman, J. Hopkins and A. Wener, 'Hyperactives as Young Adults: A Controlled Prospective Follow-up of 75 Children', *Archives of General Psychiatry*, 36 (1979), pp. 675–81; B. Greenfield, L. Hechtman and G. Weiss, 'Two Subgroups of Hyperactives as Adults: Correlations of Outcome', *Canadian Journal of Psychiatry*, 31 (1986), pp. 505–8.

31 L. Hechtman, G. Weiss, T. Perlman, 'Hyperactives as Young Adults: Past and Current Substance Abuse and Antisocial Behavior', *American Journal of Orthopsychiatry*, 54 (1984), pp. 415–25.

32 Weiss quoted in Carrey, 'Interview', p. 341.

33 Ibid.

34 G. Weiss, L. Hechtman and T. Perlman, 'Hyperactives as Young Adults: School, Employer, and Self-Rating Scales Obtained during Ten-year Follow-up Evaluation', *American Journal of Orthopsychiatry*,

48 (1978), pp. 438–45.

35 K. K. Minde and Nancy J. Cohen, 'Hyperactive Children in Canada and Uganda: A Comparative Evaluation', *Journal of the American Academy of Child Psychiatry*, 17 (1978), pp. 476–87.

36 Ibid., pp. 483–4.

37 Klaus K. Minde, 'The Hyperactive Child', *Canadian Medical Association Journal*, 112 (1975), p. 130.

38 N. J. Cohen and K. Minde, 'The "Hyperactive Syndrome" in Kindergarten: Comparison of Children with Pervasive and Situational Symptoms', *Journal of Child Psychology and Psychiatry*, 24 (1983), pp. 443–55.

39 Donald H. Sykes, Virginia I. Douglas, Gabrielle Weiss and Klaus K. Minde, 'Attention in Hyperactive Children and the Effect of Methylphenidate (Ritalin)', *Journal of Child Psychology and Psychiatry*, 12 (1971), pp. 129–39.

40 Ibid.; Donald H. Sykes, Virginia I. Douglas and Gert Morgenstern, 'The Effect of Methylphenidate (Ritalin) on Sustained Attention in Hyperactive Children', *Psychopharmacologia*, 25 (1972), pp. 262–74; V. I. Douglas, 'Stop, Look and Listen: The Problem of Sustained Attention and Impulse Control in Hyperactive and Normal Children', *Canadian Journal of Behavioural Science*, 4 (1972), pp. 259–82; Donald H. Sykes, Virginia I. Douglas and Gert Morgenstern, 'Sustained Attention in Hyperactive Children', *Journal of Child Psychology and Psychiatry*, 14 (1973), pp. 213–20.

41 J. E. Goggin, 'Sex Difference in the Activity Level of Preschool Children as a Possible Precursor of Hyperactivity', *Journal of Genetic Psychology*, 127 (1975), pp. 75–81; A. James and E. Taylor, 'Sex Differences in the Hyperkinetic Syndrome of Childhood', *Journal of Child Psychology and Psychiatry*, 31 (1990), pp. 437–46.

42 P. O. Quinn, 'Treating Adolescent Girls and Women with ADHD: Gender-specific Issues', *Journal of Clinical Psychology*, 61 (2005), pp. 579–87.

43 Ray Holland, 'Hyperactivity in Children', *Canadian Medical Association Journal*, 140 (1989), pp. 896–7.

44 Canadian Paediatric Society, 'Use of Methylphenidate for Attention Deficit Hyperactivity Disorder', *Canadian Medical Association Journal*, 142 (1990), pp. 817–18.

45 J. L. Rapoport, I. T. Lott, D. F. Alexander and A. U. Abramson,
    'Urinary Noradrenaline and Playroom Behaviour in Hyperactive
    Children', *Lancet*, 296 (1970), p. 1141.

46 Mark A. Stewart, 'Urinary Noradrenaline and Playroom Behaviour in
    Hyperactive Children', *Lancet*, 297 (1971), p. 140.

47 J.W.G. Gibb and J. F. MacMahon, 'Arrested Mental Development
    Induced by Lead-Poisoning', BMJ, 1 (1955), pp. 320–23; D. A. Pond,
    'Psychiatric Aspects of Epileptic and Brain-damaged Children', BMJ,
    2 (1961), pp. 1377–82, 1454–9; Philip Graham and Michael Rutter,
    'Organic Brain Syndrome: Child Psychiatric Disorder', BMJ, 3 (1968),
    pp. 695–700.

48 C. Ounsted, 'The Hyperkinetic Syndrome in Epileptic Children',
    Lancet, 269 (1955), pp. 303–11; T.T.S. Ingram, 'A Characteristic Form
    of Overactive Behaviour in Brain Damaged Children', *Journal of
    Mental Science*, 102 (1956), pp. 550–58; Frederick Edward Kratter,
    'The Physiognomic, Psychometric, Behavioural and Neurological
    Aspects of Phenylketonuria', *Journal of Mental Science*, 105 (1959),
    pp. 421–7.

49 Michael Knipe, '"Concentration Drug" Used in Schools', *The Times*
    (1 July 1970), p. 6; Anonymous, 'Neurology: Hyperactive Children',
    The Times (19 May 1976), p. 6; Mark Vaughan, 'Schoolchildren "Put
    on Drugs Because Class Behaviour Does Not Fit"', *The Times* (1
    December 1977), p. 5.

50 Dorothy V. M. Bishop, 'Which Neurodevelopmental Disorders Get
    Researched and Why?', PPLOS ONE, 5 (2010), e15112, at
    www.ncbi.nlm.nih.gov, accessed 27 April 2011.

51 Steven Box, 'Preface', in *The Myth of the Hyperactive Child: And Other
    Means of Child Control* (New York, [1975] 1981), pp. 17, 23.

52 Lionel Hersov quoted in Rachel Cullen, 'Should Naughty Children
    Be Drugged?', *The Times* (15 September 1981), p. 11. Resistance to
    psychopharmacology in the UK is somewhat ironic considering the
    prominent British pharmaceutical industry and the fact that a good
    deal of the world's Ritalin is produced in the UK. International
    Narcotics Control Board (INCB), *Psychotropic Substances* (Vienna,
    2009), p. 38.

53 Michael Rutter, 'Brain Damage Syndromes in Childhood: Concepts
    and Findings', *Journal of Child Psychology and Psychiatry*, 18 (1977),

p. 18. Such thinking persists today: Nicky Hart and Louba Benassaya, 'Social Deprivation or Brain Dysfunction: Data and the Discourse of ADHD in Britain and North America', in *Rethinking ADHD: From Brain to Culture*, ed. Sami Timimi and Jonathan Leo (Basingstoke, 2009), pp. 218–51.

54 Michael Rutter, J. Tizzard, W. Yule, P. Graham, T. Whitmore, 'Research Report: Isle of Wight Studies, 1964–1974', *Psychological Medicine*, 6 (1976), pp. 313–32; Michael Rutter, 'Isle of Wight Revisited: Twenty-Five Years of Child Psychiatric Epidemiology', in *Annual Progress in Child Psychiatry and Child Development*, ed. Stella Chess and Margaret E. Hertzig (New York, 1990), p. 148.

55 J. E. Oliver and A. H. Buchanan, 'Generations of Maltreated Children and Multiagency Care in One Kindred', *British Journal of Psychiatry*, 135 (1979), pp. 289–303.

56 N. Richamn and P. Graham, 'Prevalence of Behaviour Problems in 3-year-old Children', *Journal of Child Psychology and Psychiatry*, 16 (1975), p. 285.

57 Anonymous, 'Minimal Brain Dysfunction', *Lancet*, 302 (1973), p. 488.

58 Anonymous, 'Hyperactivity', *Lancet*, 312 (1978), p. 561; Box, 'Preface', pp. 17, 23–4.

59 Anonymous, 'Minimal Brain Dysfunction', pp. 487–8; Mark A. Stewart and B. H. Burne, 'Minimal Brain Dysfunction', *Lancet*, 302 (1973), p. 852.

60 Box, 'Preface', p. 24.

61 Hyperactive Children's Support Group, 'Our Publications', at www.hacsg.org.uk, accessed 27 April 2011.

62 Anonymous, 'Feingold's Regimen for Hyperkinesis', *Lancet*, 314 (1979), pp. 617–18; Trevor Fishlock, 'Lead in Petrol: Bad for Cars but Far Worse for Children's Health', *The Times* (13 December 1979), p. 15; Anonymous, 'Food Additives and Hypereactivity', *Lancet*, 319 (1982), pp. 662–3; Des Wilson, 'Petrol: Must Our Children Still Be Poisoned?', *The Times* (8 February 1982), p. 8; Suzanne Greaves, 'With Added Goodness?' *The Times* (21 August 1985), p. 11.

63 Andrew Wadge, 'Colours and Hyperactivity', at www.fsascience.net, accessed 27 April 2011. My own experience speaking to parents, health professionals and the general public in the UK and North America also suggests a much greater willingness for British people

to endorse the possibility that food additives could trigger hyperactivity.

64 WHO, *International Classification of Disease*, vol. 9 (Geneva, 1978);
    E. Taylor and S. Sandberg, 'Hyperactive Behavior in English School-
    children: A Questionnaire Survey', *Journal of Abnormal Child
    Psychology*, 12 (1984), pp. 143–56.

65 Geoffrey Thorley, 'Hyperkinetic Syndrome of Childhood: Clinical
    Characteristics', *British Journal of Psychiatry*, 144 (1984), p. 16.

66 Anonymous, 'Does Hyperactivity Matter?', *Lancet*, 327 (1986),
    pp. 73–74.

67 Eric A. Taylor, 'Childhood Hyperactivity', *British Journal of Psychiatry*,
    149 (1986), p. 570.

68 E. Taylor, R. Schachar, G. Thorley and M. Wieselberg, 'Conduct
    Disorder and Hyperactivity: 1. Separation of Hyperactivity and
    Antisocial Conduct in British Child Psychiatric Patients', *British
    Journal of Psychiatry*, 149 (1986), pp. 760–67.

69 M. Prendergast, E. Taylor, J. L. Rapoport, J. Bartlo, M. Donnelly,
    A. Zametkin, M. B. Ahearn, G. Dunn and H. M. Wieselberg, 'The
    Diagnosis of Childhood Hyperactivity: A US-UK Cross-National
    Study of DSM-II and ICD-9', *Journal of Child Psychology and Psychiatry*,
    29 (1988), p. 290; J. M. Swanson, J. A. Sergeant, E. Taylor, E.J.S.
    Sonuga-Barke, P. S. Jenson and D. P. Cantwell, 'Attention-Deficit Hy-
    peractivity Disorder and Hyperkinetic Disorder', *Lancet*, 351 (1998),
    pp. 429–33.

70 NICE, 'Attention Deficit Hyperactivity Disorder', *NICE Clinical Guide-
    line*, 72 (2008), p. 6.

71 P. Hill and E. Taylor, 'An Auditable Protocol for Treating Attention
    Deficit/Hyperactivity Disorder', *Archives of Disease in Childhood*, 84
    (2001), pp. 404–9.

72 Tracy Alloway, Julian Elliott and Jone Holmes, 'The Prevalence of
    ADHD-like Symptoms in a Community Sample', *Journal of Attention
    Disorders*, 14 (2010), pp. 52–6.

73 NICE, *Attention Deficit Hyperactivity Disorder: Diagnosis and Management
    of ADHD in Children, Young People and Adults* (London, 2009), p. 16, at
    www.nice.org.uk, accessed 2 May 2011.

74 A. Thapar, R. Harrington, K. Ross and P. McGuffin, 'Does the
    Definition of ADHD Affect Heritability?', *Journal of the American*

Academy of Child and Adolescent Psychiatry, 39 (2000), pp. 1528–36; J. Kuntsi and J. Stevenson, 'Psychological Mechanisms in Hyperactivity: II. The Role of Genetic Factors', *Journal of Child Psychology and Psychiatry*, 42 (2001), pp. 211–19.

75 NICE, *Attention Deficit Hyperactivity Disorder*, p. 34.

76 Ibid., p. 533.

77 Ibid., pp. 28–9.

78 Ibid., pp. 70–74.

79 Ibid., p. 303.

80 For a pithy account of the American approach, see Russell A. Barkley, 'International Consensus Statement on ADHD', *Clinical Child and Family Psychology Review*, 5 (2002), pp. 89–111. Although the Statement is nominally 'International', the vast majority of the signees are American.

81 INCB, *Report of the International Narcotics Control Board for 2009* (Vienna, 2009), p. 26.

82 Sami Timimi, 'Why Diagnosis of ADHD Has Increased So Rapidly in the West: A Cultural Perspective', in *Rethinking ADHD: From Brain to Culture*, ed. Sami Timimi and Jonathan Leo (Basingstoke, 2009), pp. 145–6.

83 Feinstein, *History of Autism*.

84 Sami Timimi, 'The McDonaldization of Childhood: Children's Mental Health in Neo-Liberal Cultures', *Transcultural Psychiatry*, 47 (2010), pp. 697–8.

85 Timimi and Maitra, 'ADHD and Globalization', p. 213.

86 R. J. Simmons, 'Observations of Child Psychiatry in China', *Canadian Journal of Psychiatry*, 28 (1983), pp. 124–7; Y. C. Shen, Y. F. Wang and X. L. Yang, 'An Epidemiological Investigation of Minimal Brain Dysfunction in Six Elementary Schools in Beijing', *Journal of Child Psychology and Psychiatry*, 26 (1985), pp. 777–87.

87 Timimi and Maitra, 'ADHD and Globalization', p. 211.

88 Xiao-Song Gai, Gong-Rui Lan and Xi-Ping Lui, 'A Meta-analytic Review on Treatment Effects on Attention Deficit/Hyperactivity Disorder Children in China', *Acta Psychologica Sinica*, 40 (2008), pp. 1190–96.

89 S. G. Crawford, 'Specific Learning Disabilities and Attention-Deficit Hyperactivity Disorder: Under-recognized in India', *Indian Journal of*

Medical Science, 61 (2007), pp. 637–8.

90 Jin-Pang Leung, 'Attention Deficit-Hyperactivity Disorder in Chinese
Children', in *Growing Up the Chinese Way: Chinese Child and Adolescent
Development*, ed. Sing Lau (Hong Kong, 1997), p. 221; P. Sitholey,
V. Agarwal and S. Chamoli, 'A Preliminary Study of Factors Affecting
Adherence to Medication in Clinic Children with Attention-
Deficit/Hyperactivity Disorder', *Indian Journal of Psychiatry*, 53 (2011),
pp. 41–4.

91 Claire E. Wilcox, Rachel Washburn and Vikram Patel, 'Seeking Help
for Attention Deficit Hyperactivity Disorder in Developing Countries:
A Study of Parental Explanatory Models in Goa, India', *Social Science
and Medicine*, 64 (2007), pp. 1600–10.

92 H. Zoëga, K. Furu, M. Halldórsson, P. H. Thomsen, A. Sourander
and J. E. Martikainen, 'Use of ADHD Drugs in Nordic Countries:
A Population-based Comparison Study', *Acta Psychiatrica Scandinavia*,
123 (2011), pp. 360–67; Markku Jahnukainen, 'Different Children in
Different Countries: ADHD in Canada and Finland', in *(De)Constructing
ADHD: Critical Guidance for Teachers and Teacher Educators*, ed. Linda J.
Graham (New York, 2009), p. 63.

93 Jonathan Gornall, 'Hyperactivity in Children: The Gillberg Affair',
BMJ, 335 (2007), pp. 370–73.

Conclusion: Happily Hyperactive?

1 P. S. Latham and P. H. Latham, 'Attention Deficit Hyperactivity
Disorder ADHD, Education, and the Law', NYU *Child Study Center*, 3
(1998), pp. 1–4; Peter Conrad and Deborah Potter, 'From Hyperactive
Children to ADHD Adults: Observations on the Expansion of Medical
Categories', *Social Problems*, 47 (2000), pp. 559–82.

2 Claudia Wallis, Hannah Bloch, Wendy Cole and James Willwerth,
'Attention Deficit Disorder: Life in Overdrive', *Time* (18 July 1994), at
www.time.com, accessed 10 May 2011.

3 Ibid.

4 Ibid.

5 Ibid.

6 Ibid.

7 Meredith Melnick, 'Faking It: Why Nearly 1 in 4 Adults Who Seek

Treatment Don't Have ADHD', *Time* (28 April 2011), at http://
healthland.time.com, accessed 11 May 2011; Paul Marshall, Ryan
Schroeder, Jeffrey O'Brien, Rebecca Fischer, Adam Ries, Brita Blesi
and Jessica Barker, 'Effectiveness of Symptom Validity Measures in
Identifying Cognitive and Behavioral Symptom Exaggeration in
Adult Attention Deficit Hyperactivity Disorder', *The Clinical Neuro-
psychologist*, 24 (2010), pp. 1204–37.

8 Marshal et al., 'Effectiveness of Symptom Validity', p. 1205.

9 Linda Caroll, 'Adults Who Claim to Have ADHD? 1 in 4 May be
Faking It', MSNBC.com (25 April 2011), at www.msnbc.msn.com,
accessed 11 May 2011.

10 Anjan Chatergee quoted in Melnick, 'Faking It'.

11 Adrian Goldberg, 'Unscrupulous Parents Seek ADHD Diagnoses for
Benefits', BBC News (6 February 2011), at www.bbc.co.uk, accessed
11 May 2011.

12 Rick Green and Patrick McKenna, ADD & *Loving It?!* (Totally ADD/Big
Brain Productions, 2009), see http://totallyadd.com, accessed 11 May
2011. Green and McKenna are comedians who, among other projects, acted on *The Red Green Show*, Canada's longest running comedy
series (1991–2006). Green played Bill Smith, a bumbling outdoors-
man whose madcap do-it-yourself projects, involving copious
amounts of duct tape, often end in disaster. McKenna played Harold
Green, a nerdy man-child who is the foil for his uncle, Red Green,
played by Steve Smith. Given Bill's disorderly, chaotic schemes, and
Harold's manic, clumsy and outspoken tendencies, it is likely that
their characters could have been diagnosed with ADHD. But that
would not have made for such a funny show.

13 Rick Green, 'Incurable but Treatable', at http://totallyadd.com (14
May 2010), accessed 11 May 2011.

14 Erik Piepenberg, 'Living in an ADD World: Lisa Loomer Talks about
"Distracted"', *New York Times* (4 March 2009), at http://artsbeat.
blogs.nytimes.com, accessed 11 May 2011.

15 Judith Warner, *We've Got Issues: Children and Parents in the Age of
Medication* (New York, 2010).

16 Tim Weber, 'Davos 2011: We're All Hyper-Connected – Now What?'
BBC News (29 January 2011), at www.bbc.co.uk, accessed 11 May 2011.

17 Ilina Singh has examined this issue from a sociological perspective.

For example, Ilina Singh, 'Will The "Real Boy" Please Behave: Dosing Dilemmas for Parents of Boys with ADHD', *American Journal of Bioethics*, 5 (2005), pp. 34–47.

18 Marcus Weaver-Hightower, 'The "Boy Turn" in Research on Gender and Education', *Review of Educational Research*, 73 (2003), pp. 471–98.

19 Kimberly A. Bazar, Anthony J. Yun, Patrick Y. Lee, Stephanie M. Daniel and John D. Doux, 'Obesity and ADHD May Represent Different Manifestations of a Common Environmental Over-sampling Syndrome: A Model for Revealing Mechanistic Overlap among Cognitive, Metabolic, and Inflammatory Disorders', *Medical Hypotheses*, 66 (2006), pp. 263–9; Sherry L. Pagoto, Carol Curtin, Stephanie C. Lemon, Linda G. Bandini, Kristin L. Schneider, Jamie S. Bodenlos and Yunsheng Ma, 'Association between Adult Attention Deficit/Hyperactivity Disorder and Obesity in the US Population', *Obesity*, 17 (2009), pp. 539–44.

20 Anonymous, 'Treadmills Put N.B. Students on Learning Track', CBC News, at www.cbc.ca, accessed 12 May 2011.

21 Richard Louv, *Last Child in the Woods: Saving Our Children from Nature Deficit Disorder* (Chapel Hill, NC, 2005).

22 See www.bluegym.org.uk, accessed 13 May 2011.

23 Sheila Riddell, Jean Kane, Gwynedd Lloyd, Gillean McCluskey, Joan Stead and Elisabet Weedon, 'School Discipline and ADHD: Are Restorative Practices the Answer?' in *(De)constructing ADHD: Critical Guidance for Teachers and Teacher Educators*, ed. Linda J. Graham (New York, 2009), pp. 187–204.

24 Sheila M. Rothman and David J. Rothman, *The Pursuit of Perfection: The Promise and Perils of Medical Enhancement* (New York, 2003).

25 Keith Wailoo, 'Old Story, Updated: Better Living Through Pills', *New York Times* (13 November 2007), at www.nytimes.com, accessed 12 May 2011.

26 Jonathan Abrams, 'Kaman Recalls Childhood Frustrations', *Los Angeles Times*, 15 January 2008.

Select Bibliography

Anderson, Camilla, *Society Pays the High Cost of Minimal Brain Damage in America* (New York, 1972)

Apple, Rima D., *Perfect Motherhood: Science and Childrearing in America* (New Brunswick, NJ, 2006)

Barkley, Russell, *Attention-deficit Hyperactivity Disorder: A Handbook for Diagnosis and Treatment*, 3rd edn (New York, 2006)

Bernstein, Irving, *Promises Kept: John F. Kennedy's New Frontier* (New York, 1991)

Bradley, Charles, 'The Behavior of Children Receiving Benzedrine', *American Journal of Psychiatry*, 94 (1937), pp. 577–85

—, 'Benzedrine and Dexedrine in the Treatment of Children's Behavior Disorders', *Pediatrics*, 5 (1950), pp. 24–37

Brancaccio, Maria Teresa, 'Educational Hyperactivity: The Historical Emergence of a Concept', *Intercultural Education*, 11 (2000), pp. 165–77

Breggin, Peter, *Talking Back to Ritalin: What Doctors Aren't Telling You about Stimulants for Children* (Monroe, ME, 1998)

Brumberg, Joan Jacobs, *Fasting Girls: The History of Anorexia Nervosa* (Cambridge, MA, 1989)

Clouston, Thomas S., 'Stages of Overexcitability, Hypersensitiveness and Mental Explosiveness and Their Treatment by the Bromides', *Scottish Medical and Surgical Journal*, 4 (1899), pp. 481–90

Collins, Harry, and Trevor Pinch, *Dr Golem: How to Think About Medicine* (Chicago, IL, 2005)

Conant, James Bryant, *The American High School Today: A First Report to Interested Citizens* (New York, 1959)

—, *Slums and Suburbs* (New York, 1961)

Conners, C. Keith, *Food Additives and Hyperactive Children* (New York, 1980)

—, *Feeding the Brain: How Foods Affect Children* (New York, 1989)

Conners, C. Keith, and Leon Eisenberg, 'The Effects of Methylphenidate on Symptomology and Learning in Disturbed Children', *American Journal of Psychiatry*, 120 (1963), pp. 458–64

Conrad, Peter, 'The Discovery of Hyperkinesis: Notes on the Medicalization of Deviant Behavior', *Social Problems*, 23 (1975), pp. 12–21

—, *Identifying Hyperactive Children: The Medicalization of Deviant Behavior* (Toronto, 1976)

Conrad, Peter, and Deborah Potter, 'From Hyperactive Children to ADHD Adults: Observations on the Expansion of Medical Categories', *Social Problems*, 47 (2000), pp. 559–82

Cooter, Roger, ed., *In the Name of the Child: Health and Welfare, 1880–1940* (London, 1992)

Crichton, Alexander, *An Inquiry into the Nature and Origin of Mental Derangement Comprehending a Concise System of the Physiology and Pathology of the Human Mind and a History of the Passions and their Effects* (London, 1798)

DeGrandpre, Richard, *Ritalin Nation: Rapid-fire Culture and the Transformation of Human Consciousness* (New York, 1999)

Diller, Lawrence, 'The Run on Ritalin: Attention Deficit Disorder and Stimulant Treatment in the 1990s', *Hastings Center Report*, 26 (1996), pp. 12–18

Dyck, Erika, *Psychedelic Psychiatry: LSD from Clinic to Campus* (Baltimore, MD, 2008)

Dyck, Erika, and Christopher Fletcher, eds, *Locating Health: Historical and Anthropological Investigations of Place and Health* (London, 2010)

Ehrenreich, Barbara, and Deirdre English, *For Her Own Good: 150 Years of the Experts' Advice to Women* (Garden City, NY, 1979)

Feingold, Ben F., *Why Your Child is Hyperactive* (New York, 1974)

Fleck, Ludwik, *Genesis and Development of a Scientific Fact* [1935] (Chicago, IL, 1979)

Foucault, Michel, *Madness and Civilization: A History of Insanity in the Age of Reason*, trans. Richard Howard (New York, 1965)

Freud, Anna, *Normality and Pathology in Childhood* (New York, 1965)

Garber, Stephen W., Marianne Daniels Garber and Robyn Freedman Spizman, *Beyond Ritalin: Facts about Medication and Other Strategies for Helping Children, Adolescents, and Adults with Attention Deficit Disorder*

(New York, 1996)

Gittins, Diana, *The Child in Question* (London, 1998)

Grinspoon, Lester, and Peter Hedblom, *Speed Culture: Amphetamine Use and Abuse in America* (Cambridge, MA, 1975)

Grob, Gerald N., *From Asylum to Community: Mental Health Policy in Modern America*, (Princeton, NJ, 1991)

—, *The Mad among Us: A History of the Care of America's Mentally Ill* (New York, 1994)

Gutek, Gerald L., *Education in the United States: An Historical Perspective* (Englewood Cliffs, NJ, 1986)

Hacking, Ian, 'Making up People', in *The Science Studies Reader*, ed. Mario Biagioli (New York, 1999), 161–71

Haggett, Ali, *Desperate Housewives, Neuroses and the Domestic Environment, 1945–1970* (London, 2012)

Hale, Nathan G., *The Rise and Crisis of Psychoanalysis in the United States* (Oxford, 1995)

Hartmann, Thom, *Attention Deficit Disorder: A Different Perception* (Grass Valley, CA, 1997)

Hayes, Sarah, 'Rabbits and Rebels: The Medicalization of Maladjusted Children in Mid-twentieth Century Britain', in *Health and the Modern Home*, ed. Mark Jackson (New York, 2007), pp. 128–52

Healy, David, *The Antidepressant Era* (Cambridge, MA, 1997)

—, *Let Them Eat Prozac: The Unhealthy Relationship between the Pharmaceutical Industry and Depression* (New York, 2004)

—, *Mania: A Short History of Bipolar Disorder* (Baltimore, MD, 2008)

Hendrick, Harry, *Child Welfare: Historical Dimensions, Contemporary Debate* (Bristol, 2003)

Herzberg, David, *Happy Pills in America: From Miltown to Prozac* (Baltimore, MD, 2009)

Hoffmann, Heinrich, *Struwwelpeter: Merry Stories and Funny Pictures* (New York, [1844] 1848), at http://www.gutenberg.org

Horwitz, Allan V., *Creating Mental Illness* (Chicago, IL, 2003)

Iversen, Leslie, *Speed, Ecstasy, Ritalin: The Science of Amphetamines* (Oxford, [2006] 2008)

Jackson, Mark, *The Borderland of Imbecility: Medicine, Society and the Fabrication of the Feeble Mind in Late Victorian and Edwardian England* (Manchester, 2000)

Joint Commission on the Mental Health of Children, *Social Change and the Mental Health of Children* (New York, 1973)

Jones, Kathleen W., *Taming the Troublesome Child: American Families, Child Guidance, and the Limits of Psychiatric Authority* (Cambridge, MA, 1999)

Kanner, Leo, *Child Psychiatry*, 3rd edn (Springfield, IL, 1957)

Kennedy, John F., 'Message from the President of the United States Relative to Mental Illness and Mental Retardation', *American Journal of Psychiatry*, 120 (1963/4), pp. 729–37

Kuhn, Thomas, *The Structure of Scientific Revolutions*, 3rd edn (Chicago, IL, [1962] 1996)

Kutchins, Herb, and Stuart A. Kirk, *Making Us Crazy: DSM – The Psychiatric Bible and the Creation of Mental Disorders* (New York, 1997)

Lakoff, Andrew, 'Adaptive Will: The Evolution of Attention Deficit Disorder', *Journal of the History of the Behavioral Sciences*, 36 (2000), pp. 149–69

Laufer, Maurice W., and Eric Denhoff, 'Hyperkinetic Behavior Syndrome in Children', *Journal of Pediatrics*, 50 (1957), pp. 463–74

Laufer, Maurice W., Eric Denhoff and Gerald Solomons, 'Hyperkinetic Impulse Disorder in Children's Behavior Problems', *Psychosomatic Medicine*, 19 (1957), pp. 38–49

Löwy, Ilana, 'The Strength of Loose Concepts – Boundary Concepts, Federative Experimental Strategies and Disciplinary Growth: The Case of Immunology', *History of Science*, 30 (1992), pp. 371–96

Mackarness, Richard, *Not All in the Mind: How Unsuspected Food Allergy Can Affect Your Body AND Your Mind* (London, 1976)

Marland, Hilary, and Marijke Gijswijt-Hofsra, eds, *Cultures of Child Health in Britain and the Netherlands in the Twentieth Century* (Amsterdam, 2003)

Maté, Gabor, *Scattered Minds: A New Look at the Origins and Healing of Attention Deficit Disorder* (Toronto, 1999)

Mayes, Rick, and Adam Rafalovich, 'Suffer the Restless Children: The Evolution of ADHD and Paediatric Stimulant Use, 1900–1980', *History of Psychiatry*, 18 (2007), pp. 435–57

Metzl, Jonathan Michel, *Prozac on the Couch: Prescribing Gender in the Era of Wonder Drugs* (Durham, NC, 2003)

Mezzich, Juan E., Arthur Kleinman, Horacio Fabrega, Jr, and Delores L. Parron, eds, *Culture and Psychiatric Diagnosis: A DSM-IV Perspective* (Washington, DC, 1996)

Micale, Mark S., *Approaching Hysteria: Disease and Its Interpretations* (Princeton, NJ, 1995)

Mintz, Steven, and Susan Kellogg, *Domestic Revolutions: A Social History of Family Life* (New York, 1988)

Modée, Steven A., 'Post Sputnik Panic', *English Journal*, 69 (1980), p. 56

Moon, Nathan William, 'The Amphetamine Years: A Study of the Medical Applications and Extramedical Consumption of Psychostimulant Drugs in the Postwar United States, 1945–1980', PhD thesis, Georgia Tech University, 2009

Owram, Doug, *Born at the Right Time: A History of the Baby-boom Generation* (Toronto, 1996)

Porter, Roy, *The Greatest Benefit to Mankind: A Medical History of Humanity from Antiquity to the Present* (London, 1999)

Porter, Roy, and Mark S. Micale, eds, *Discovering the History of Psychiatry* (Oxford, 1994)

Prescott, Heather Munro, *A Doctor of Their Own: The History of Adolescent Medicine* (Cambridge, MA, 1998)

Pressman, Jack D., *Last Resort: Psychosurgery and the Limits of Medicine* (Cambridge, 1998)

Rafalovich, Adam, 'The Conceptual History of Attention-deficit/Hyperactivity Disorder: Idiocy, Imbecility, Encephalitis, and the Child Deviant, 1877–1929', *Deviant Behavior*, 22 (2001), pp. 93–115

—, 'Disciplining Domesticity: Framing the ADHD Parent and Child', *The Sociological Quarterly*, 42 (2001), pp. 373–93

—, *Framing ADHD Children: A Critical Examination of the History, Discourse, and Everyday Experience of Attention Deficit/Hyperactivity Disorder* (Lanham, MD, 2004)

Rafferty, Max, *Suffer, Little Children* (New York, 1963)

Randolph, Theron G., and Ralph W. Moss, *An Alternative Approach to Allergies: The New Field of Clinical Ecology Unravels the Environmental Causes of Mental and Physical Ills* (New York, 1980)

Rapp, Doris J., *Allergies and the Hyperactive Child* (New York, 1979)

Rasmussen, Nicolas, *On Speed: The Many Lives of Amphetamine* (New York, 2008)

Ravitch, Diane, *The Troubled Crusade: American Education, 1945–1980* (New York, 1983)

Rickover, Hyman G., *American Education – A National Failure: The Problem of*

Our Schools and What We Can Learn from England (New York, 1963)

Rippa, S. Alexander, *Education in a Free Society: An American History*, 7th edn (New York, 1992)

Rosenberg, Charles E., *Explaining Epidemics and Other Studies in the History of Medicine* (Cambridge, 1992)

Ross, Dorothea M., and Sheila A. Ross, *Hyperactivity: Research, Theory, and Action* (New York, 1976)

Rothman, Sheila M., and David J. Rothman, *The Pursuit of Perfection: The Promise and Perils of Medical Enhancement* (New York, 2003)

Rutter, Michael J. Tizzard, W. Yule, P. Graham, T. Whitmore, 'Research Report: Isle of Wight Studies, 1964–1974', *Psychological Medicine*, 6 (1976), pp. 313–32

Sandberg, Seija, and Joanne Barton, 'Historical Development', in *Hyperactivity and Attention Disorders of Childhood*, ed. Seija Sandberg (Cambridge, 2002), pp. 1–29.

Schrag, Peter, and Diane Divoky, *The Myth of the Hyperactive Child: And Other Means of Child Control* (New York, [1975] 1982)

Shorter, Edward, *From Paralysis to Fatigue: A History of Psychosomatic Illness in the Modern Era* (New York, 1992)

—, *A History of Psychiatry* (New York, 1997)

—, *Before Prozac: The Troubled History of Mood Disorders in Psychiatry* (Oxford, 2009)

Silbergeld, E. K., and A. M. Goldberg, 'Hyperactivity: A Lead-induced Behavior Disorder', *Environmental Health Perspectives*, 7 (1974), pp. 227–32

Singh, Ilina, 'Bad Boys, Good Mothers, and the "Miracle" of Ritalin, *Science in Context*, 15 (2002), pp. 577–603.

—, 'Biology in Context: Social and Cultural Perspectives on ADHD, *Children & Society*, 16 (2002), pp. 360–67

—, 'Boys Will Be Boys: Fathers' Perspectives on ADHD Symptoms, Diagnosis, and Drug Treatment', *Harvard Review of Psychiatry*, 11 (2003), pp. 308–16

—, 'Doing Their Jobs: Mothering with Ritalin in a Culture of Mother-blame', *Social Science & Medicine*, 59 (2004), pp. 1193–1205

—, 'Will The "Real Boy" Please Behave: Dosing Dilemmas for Parents of Boys with ADHD', *American Journal of Bioethics*, 5 (2005), pp. 34–47

Singh, Ilina, and Kelly Kelleher, 'Neuroenhancement in Young People:

Proposal for Research, Policy, and Clinical Management', AJOB
Neuroscience, 1 (2010), pp. 3–16

Smith, Matthew, 'Psychiatry Limited: Hyperactivity and the Evolution of
American Psychiatry, 1957–1980', Social History of Medicine, 21 (2008),
pp. 541–59

—, 'The Uses and Abuses of the History of Hyperactivity', in
(De)Constructing ADHD: Critical Guidance for Teachers and Teacher Educators,
ed. Linda J. Graham (New York, 2010)

—, 'A Place for Hyperactivity: Sputnik, the Cold War "Brain Race" and the
Origins of Hyperactivity in the United States, 1957–1968', in Locating
Health, ed. Erika Dyck and Christopher Fletcher (London, 2011)

—, An Alternative History of Hyperactivity: Food Additives and the Feingold Diet
(New Brunswick, NJ, 2011)

Spring, Joel, The American School, 1642–1990: Varieties of Historical Interpretation of the Foundations and Development of American Education, 2nd
edn (White Plains, NY, 1990)

Stewart, John, 'The Scientific Claims of British Child Guidance, 1918–
1945', British Journal for the History of Science, 42 (2009), pp. 407–32

Still, George F., 'The Goulstonian Lectures on Some Abnormal Psychical
Conditions in Children', Lancet, 159 (1902), pp. 1008–12; 1077–82;
1163–8

Thomson, Mathew, Psychological Subjects: Identity, Culture and Health in
Twentieth-century Britain (Oxford, 2009)

Timimi, Sami, Naughty Boys: Anti-social Behaviour, ADHD and the Role of
Culture (New York, 2005)

Timimi, Sami, and Begum Maitra, eds, Critical Voices in Child and Adolescent
Mental Health (London, 2006)

Timimi, Sami, and Jonathan Leo, eds, Rethinking ADHD: From Brain to
Culture (Basingstoke, 2009)

Tone, Andrea, 'Listening to the Past: Psychiatry, History, and Anxiety',
Canadian Journal of Psychiatry, 50 (2005), pp. 373–80

—, The Age of Anxiety: A History of America's Turbulent Affair with Tranquilizers
(New York, 2009)

Welshman, John, From Transmitted Deprivation to Social Exclusion: Policy,
Poverty and Parenting (Bristol, 2007)

Wender, Paul H., Minimal Brain Dysfunction in Children (New York, 1971)

Winchell, Carol Ann, The Hyperkinetic Child: A Bibliography of Medical,

Educational, and Behavioral Studies (Greenwood, CT, 1975)

Young, Allan, *The Harmony of Illusions: Inventing Post-traumatic Stress Disorder* (Princeton, NJ, 1995)

Zipes, Jack, *Sticks and Stones: The Troublesome Success of Children's Literature from Slovenly Peter to Harry Potter* (New York, 2002)

Acknowledgements

This project began during an MA seminar run by Julian Martin at the University of Alberta. It was then, probably on a bitter November afternoon, that I began thinking about hyperactivity from a historical perspective and I thank Professor Martin for challenging me to do so. Others at the U of A also deserve thanks, particularly the legendary David Wangler and Lesley Cormack, both of whom gave me the confidence I often lacked. I also received support and guidance from Pat Prestwich, Susan L. Smith, Erika Dyck, Matthew Eisler and Greg Anderson.

Many friends from my time as a career counsellor also deserve acknowledgement. Countless Friday evenings were spent commiserating with Terry Luhoway, Wendy Marusin, Philipa Hardy, Trevor April, Janelle Beblow, Sharon Brown and others at Chateau Louis about how to help troubled kids succeed despite the byzantine provincial bureaucracy. Thanks also to Brian Mader for his kindness and encouragement.

At Exeter I received exemplary supervision, guidance and support by Mark Jackson at the Centre for Medical History. Claire Keyte and Mary Carter were indispensible, as were Mark Doidge, Matthias Reiss, Rowan Fraser, Kiu Yu, Claude Kananack, Sharon Marshall, Ed Ramsden, Isabelle Charmantier, Ali Haggett, Sarah Hayes, Debbie Palmer, Pamela Dale, Pamela Richardson, Tindy Agaba and JJ Reilly.

Thanks to the University of Strathclyde for offering me a job. I will do my utmost to ensure that they do not regret it! Thanks especially to colleagues at CSHHH for their warm Glasgow welcome, particularly, Jim Mills, Arthur McIvor, Emma Newlands and John Stewart.

My research has relied enormously on the financial support, training and resources of the Wellcome Trust, and the encouragement of Tony Woods, Nils Fietje, Ross MacFarlane, Phoebe Harkins and others. Because of the Wellcome Trust, associations such as the Society for the Social History of Medicine, and the vibrant medical history community, the UK is a wonderful place to study the history of medicine. I am also profoundly grateful for the support of Vivian Constantinopoulos at Reaktion. I met Vivian at one of Jeremy Black's book launches, so thanks for the invitation, Jeremy!

Finally, my family and friends deserve immeasurable thanks for persevering with me through what has been a meandering career path. I will always be indebted to Michelle, Dashiell, Mom, Dad, Liz, Jeremy, Addison, Kellan, the Burkes, Alice and all my family and friends in Canada.

Index

243